MALIGNANT MESOTHELIOMA

Edited by **Carmen Belli** and **Santosh Anand**

Malignant Mesothelioma

http://dx.doi.org/10.5772/1648
Edited by Carmen Belli and Santosh Anand

Contributors

James I. Phillips, David Rees, Jill Murray, John C.A. Davies, Yasumitsu Nishimura, Megumi Maeda, Naoko Kumagai-Takei, Hidenori Matsuzaki, Suni Lee, Kazuya Fukuoka, Takashi Nakano, Takumi Kishimoto, Takemi Otsuki, Loredana Albonici, Camilla Palumbo, Vittorio Manzari, Rossella Galati, Giulia Pasello, Adolfo Favaretto

Published by InTech

Janeza Trdine 9, 51000 Rijeka, Croatia

Publishing Process Manager Sandra Bakic
Technical Editor InTech DTP team
Cover InTech Design team

Additional hard copies can be obtained from orders@intechopen.com

Malignant Mesothelioma, Edited by Carmen Belli and Santosh Anand
p. cm.
ISBN 978-953-51-0901-3

For EU product safety concerns:
IN TECH d.o.o., Prolaz Marije Krucifikse Kozulić 3, 51000 Rijeka, Croatia,
info@intechopen.com or visit our website at intechopen.com.

Meet the editors

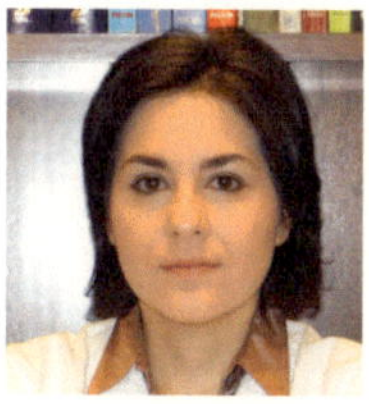

Dr. Carmen Belli (MD., PhD.) is an oncologist working at San Raffaele Hospital in Milan, Italy. She has been actively involved in the clinical research with particular focus on mesothelioma, lung cancer, pancreatic and breast cancer. She collaborated with Italian Mesothelioma Group (Gi.Me) and had been an advisor to Buzzi Foundation in drafting research projects and clinical trials on malignant mesothelioma. She also wrote a chapter titled "Mesotelioma Pleurico (Pleural Mesothelioma)" in the book "Medicina Interna Sistematica" of Claudio Rugarli (Elsevier/Masson, 6th Ed.), a standard text-book for the students of Internal Medicine in Italy. Recently, she is more focused on pancreatic cancer and is particularly involved in studying the role of diabetic condition and hyperinsulinism in progression of pancreatic tumors. She is also following several clinical trials testing new drugs in pancreatic cancer, alone or in combination with chemotherapy.

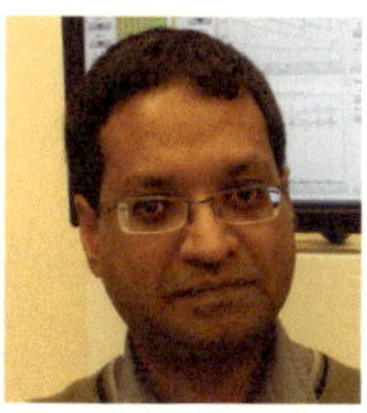

Santosh Anand (MSc.) is a senior bioinformatician at San Raffaele Scientific Institute in Milan, Italy. He has double Master's degree in Physics (IIT Kanpur, India) and in Computer Science (University of Nice, France), respectively, and has extensive experience in interdisciplinary and translational research. His main research interest is in integration and analysis of different kinds of biological data (genomics, proteomics, NGS) to understand the molecular basis of genetic diseases. He is particularly interested in biomarker studies and has worked on biomarkers for lung cancer, fabry disease and pancreatic cancer. Currently he is involved in several clinical and basic research projects in type-I diabetes (T1D). These include finding ways to increase the efficacy of bone marrow islet transplant (in T1D pts.) and (pre-clinical) stem cell therapy; and dissecting the roles of neutrophil, Teff and Treg cells in T1D. In the past, he worked as bioinformatician at Telethon Institute of Genetics and Medicine (Naples, Italy) and managed and analyzed all the data of EU integrated project EURExpress.

Contents

Preface

Malignant mesothelioma (MM) is a highly invasive tumor arising from the mesothelial cells of serosal surfaces. It shows an extremely poor progression and is diagnosed mostly in locally advanced or metastatic stage, thus drastically limiting its treatment options. Past asbestos exposure has been shown to be the most important predictor of MM, although other environmental and genetic factors like Simian Virus-40 (SV-40) infection and genetic predisposition might also play important roles.

This book brings together the knowledge of experts in the filed of malignant mesothelioma who provide their invaluable insights into this deadly disease from different perspectives.

The book starts with a *tour de force* account of MM epidemiology in South Africa (SA) by scholars who have spent major part of their professional careers working in this field. In a gripping *tell-a-tale,* they recall how South Africa benefitted financially from the exploitation of its asbestos mineral reserves, but at a huge cost of human lives due to asbestos related diseases, including MM and lung cancer. South Africa plays a historically important role in our understanding of epidemiology of MM, thanks mainly to the seminal work by Dr. J. C. Wagner who showed definitive link between asbestos exposure and mesothelioma. In this chapter, the authors give a detailed account of the cases of mesothelioma in South Africa meticulously linking them to different forms of asbestos exposure (both occupational and non-occupational). They further dissect the carcinogenic potentials of the most common asbestos fibers mined in SA. There are many important lessons to be learnt from this SA experience, aptly summarized at the end of this chapter.

In the next chapter, Yasumitsu Nishimura et al. describe in detail the anti-tumor immunity and immunological alterations in MM, a hitherto neglected but nevertheless important aspect of MM-geneis. The authors show that exposure to asbestos might cause a suppressive effect on anti-tumor immunity in addition to the tumorigenic effect on mesothelial cells. This 'immunological' insight could not have come at a better time as only recently it is shown that blockade of PD-1, an inhibitory receptor expressed by T cells, gives promising therapeutic results in patients of many advanced cancers (Suzanne L. Topalian et al., and Julie R. Brahmer et al.; NEJM, 2012).

In the following chapter, Loredana Albonici and colleagues describe the roles of inflammation and angiogenic growth factors in MM. Angiogenesis plays a key role in the growth of any tumor as shown by the seminal work of Judah Folkman in 1971. Here the authors go beyond this basic fact by showing that asbestos driven inflammation plays an important role in MM and that there is a cross-talk between inflammation and angiogenesis in the genesis and progression of MM. They describe how mesothelial cells work as sentinels sensing a variety of signals and stimuli, including asbestos fibers. In response, the mesothelial cells can release a host of chemokines, cytokines and reactive oxygen and nitrogen species, thus triggering chronic inflammatory reactions potentially leading to MM. The authors show in great details the roles of various transcription factors like NF-kB, AP-1 and NFAT in this process. Furthermore, they also explore the roles of various angiogenic growth factors, many of which could be potential targets for therapy.

The penultimate chapter by Rossella Galati links the inflammation in MM to up-regulation of the inducible cyclooxygenase-2 (COX-2), leading to an increase in its product prostaglandin-E2 (PGE-2), which in turn is associated with increased risk of cancers. The author describes the complex interaction between COX-2, EGFR and Aromatase (CYP19A1), which has the potential to open new therapeutics in MM.

The last chapter by Giulia Pasello and Adolfo Favaretto describes neoadjuvant chemotherapy in malignant pleural mesothelioma (MPM). In this deadly malignancy that is refractory to almost all treatments, the possibility to pursue novel and rational strategies is extremely exciting. The chapter begins with the rationale of neoadjuvant therapy, followed by the current path to neoadjuvant chemotherapy in MPM. It culminates in an extensive review of various neoadjuvant chemotherapeutic regimens and strategies in MPM.

We would like to thank all the contributing authors for making this book possible. Our special thanks goes to publishing process managers Ms. Sandra Bakic, Ms. Martina Blecic and Mr. Vedran Greblo for their continuous help during the entire process. We would like to dedicate this book to the readers in the hope that they will find it useful in the ultimate quest for the cure of malignant mesothelioma.

Carmen Belli and Santosh Anand
San Raffaele Hospital, and San Raffaele Scientific Institute, Milan, Italy

Chapter 1

Mineralogy and Malignant Mesothelioma: The South African Experience

James I. Phillips, David Rees, Jill Murray and John C.A. Davies

Additional information is available at the end of the chapter

http://dx.doi.org/10.5772/47974

1. Introduction

South Africa is a uniquely mineral rich country. Of the six types of asbestiform minerals found in the country, three, namely crocidolite, amosite and chrysotile were mined and milled on a large commercial scale. Asbestos was used locally in South Africa, but the majority of its production was exported worldwide. In the 1970s, South Africa was the world's third largest producer of asbestos, behind Canada and the USSR. About 97% of the world's production of crocidolite and virtually all of the amosite came from South Africa.

The output from the South African asbestos mining industry peaked at 380,000 tonnes in 1977 and declined thereafter as export markets declined due to restrictive legislation in countries that imported asbestos (Virta, 2006; Kielkowski et al., 2011). Legislation in South Africa banning the use of all types of asbestos came into effect in 2008, well after the last asbestos mine ceased production in 2001 and closed in 2002. Although South Africa benefitted financially from the exploitation of its asbestos mineral reserves, the revenue from asbestos never accounted for more than 3% of the value of its total minerals output (McCulloch, 2003). There is however a high price to pay in terms of a legacy of disease and environmental contamination through mining activities and the transport of asbestos and asbestos containing products.

This account records, in the main, work done in Johannesburg at the National Institute for Occupational Health (NIOH) - formerly the Pneumoconiosis Research Unit (PRU), thereafter, the National Research Institute for Occupational Diseases and later the National Centre for Occupational Health - at the Medical Bureau for Occupational Diseases and its Division of Epidemiology Research. All the authors have spent the major part of their professional careers working at the NIOH.

All types of asbestos are crystalline silicates. Chrysotile, known locally in South Africa as white asbestos, occurs in ultramafic rock formations. It is a hydrated magnesium silicate and differs from the other types of asbestos in that it has serpentine fibres and contains only the one cation: magnesium. The other types of asbestos have straight fibres and are called amphiboles. The amphiboles all contain iron and combinations of other cations – sodium, magnesium and calcium. Crocidolite, also known as Riebeckite and locally as blue asbestos, occurs in banded ironstone formations. It contains the cations sodium, magnesium and iron. Amosite (an acronym for Asbestos Mines of South Africa), also known as Grunerite and locally as brown asbestos, occurs in banded ironstone. It contains the cations magnesium and iron. Because of their different chemical composition and crystalline structure, the different types of asbestos have different physical properties. Commercially they were used for different purposes. Chrysotile was preferred for manufacturing friction linings, asbestos cement, textiles, ropes and yarns. Amosite was used where long fibres were required. It is much more resistant to acids and sea-water than chrysotile. In compacted form it was applied as a covering for marine turbines and jet engines. It was also used in blanket form for insulation in high temperature applications. Crocidolite has a high tensile strength and was used as insulation from very high temperatures. Long crocidolite fibres were used for boiler lagging, acid resistant packings and gaskets. Short crocidolite fibres were used in the manufacture of asbestos cement (Hart, 1988). It might be expected that different types of asbestos with different chemical and physical properties would have different potentials to cause disease.

The diseases most firmly attributed to exposure to asbestos are asbestosis, pleural effusions, diffuse pleural fibrosis, pleural plaques, lung cancer and mesothelioma (Figure 1). In South Africa, asbestosis was described as early as 1928 in lung tissue sent to the South African Institute for Medical Research in Johannesburg, for examination. The tissue was obtained at autopsy from asbestos miners who worked in Southern Rhodesia, now known as Zimbabwe (Simson, 1928). The association between mesothelioma and exposure to crocidolite asbestos was published by Wagner, Sleggs and Marchand in 1960 (Wagner et al., 1960). Wagner worked at the NIOH, which was known at that time as the PRU. He was recruited by his brother in law, Ian Webster, who encouraged him to research the adverse health effects of asbestos. Despite the knowledge that inhalation of asbestos fibres could cause disease, exposure levels for miners and millers were poorly controlled (Slade, 1931). Tens of thousands of formally employed miners and millers were exposed to asbestos (McCulloch, 2003). Many workers, including women and juveniles were employed informally by the mines and there are scant if any records of these employees (McCulloch, 2002). In addition, whole communities next to mines were environmentally exposed (Abratt et al., 2004) and in some instances this exposure continues. South Africans in the manufacturing industries were exposed along with artisans such as boiler makers. Asbestos and asbestos products were used on mines that mine other commodities such as gold. In a study of 18 cases of mesothelioma occurring in gold mine workers, 15 were artisans and included boiler makers, fitters, electricians, a plumber and a mason who lined furnaces with asbestos (Davies et al., 1987). Because of the extensive use of building materials that contain asbestos (Phillips et al., 2007) (Figure 2), workers in the construction, renovation and demolition sectors have a potential risk of exposure to asbestos through their work (Figure 3).

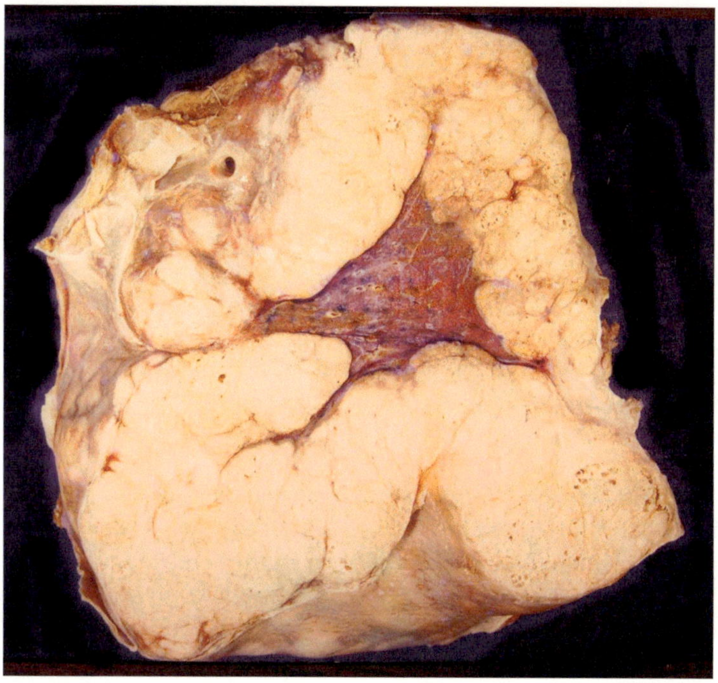

Figure 1. Gross specimen of malignant mesothelioma of the pleura. (Courtesy of NIOH archive).

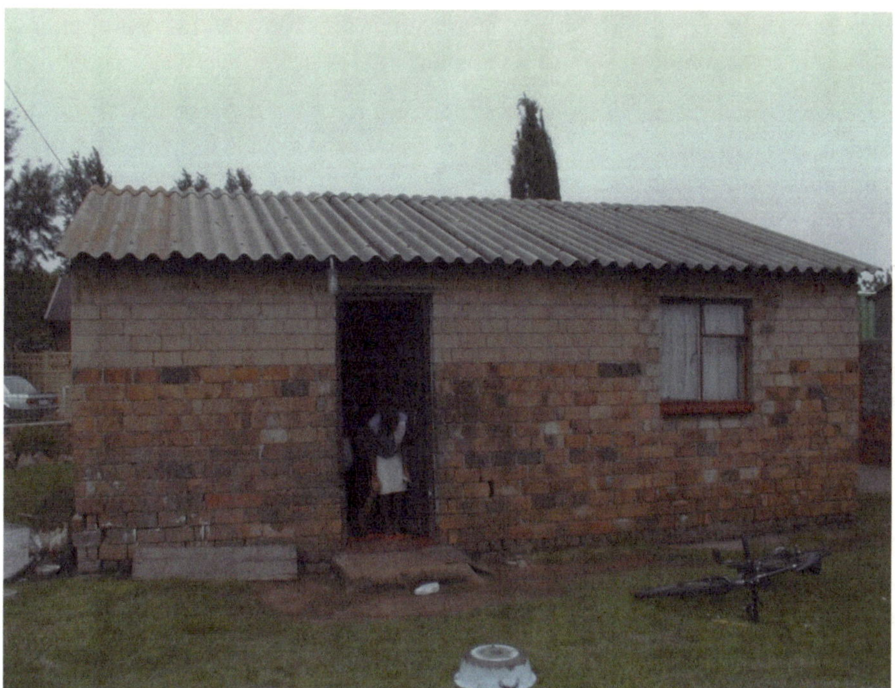

Figure 2. Typical house in Soweto near Johannesburg built circa 1960 with an asbestos cement roof. (Courtesy of Professor JI Phillips).

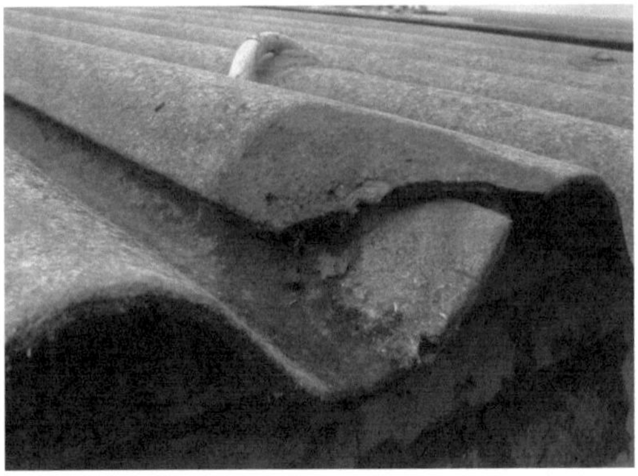

Figure 3. Detail of asbestos roof sheet in Soweto, showing damage and exposed asbestos fibres. (Courtesy of Professor JI Phillips).

Although trends in mortality due to mesothelioma in the general population have been documented in other countries (Hodgson et al., 2005; Nishikawa et al., 2008), only two South African studies have quantified the burden of asbestos-related cancers in the general population. From 1976 to 1984, estimated incidence rates for mesothelioma averaged over this period were amongst the highest for a general population anywhere in the world. For white, mixed race and black men, the standardized incidence rates for mesothelioma per million population per year aged 15 and over were calculated to be 32.9, 24.8 and 7.6 respectively and 8.9, 13.9, and 3.0 for white, mixed race and black women respectively (Zwi et al., 1989). These figures reflect predominantly occupational exposure in men and predominantly environmental exposure in women.

Mesothelioma mortality rates in the general population of South Africa have been calculated from 1995 to 2007. The age adjusted mortality rates remained stable for the period and ranged from 11 to 16 per million per-year for men and 3 to 5 per million per year for women. The data for this study were not broken down into racial groups and are therefore not directly comparable to the 1976 to 1984 study. However, rates for the period 1995 to 2007 appear to be much lower than expected. The reasons for this are not entirely clear. It may be due to under reporting or to competing causes of death relating to the AIDS epidemic in the country (Kielkowski et al., 2011).

There has been a debate that apart from asbestos a virus may be involved in the development of mesothelioma. There has been research into the association of Simian Virus 40 (SV40) and mesothelioma. SV40 was a contaminant of poliomyelitis vaccine grown on cell lines derived from Macaques and was inadvertently administered with the vaccine to many people around the world. South Africa, however, produced its own poliomyelitis vaccine which was grown in vervet monkey kidney cell cultures. Unlike Macaques, vervet monkeys (*Cercopithecus aethiops*) are not a natural host for SV40 and South African vaccines were not contaminated (Malherbe, 1974). Studies on tissue from South African cases of mesothelioma showed no evidence for an etiologic role for SV40 (Manfredi et al., 2005).

The South African experience is of three commercially important asbestos types: crocidolite, amosite and chrysotile. These will be discussed separately in order to set out in detail what is known about the role of each of these fibres in the causation of mesothelioma in South Africa.

In South Africa, crocidolite mining began in 1893, near the town of Prieska, in what was called the North Western Cape and is now known as the Northern Cape Province (McCulloch, 2003) (Figure 4). The asbestos deposits occur along a 450 kilometre line between just south of Prieska to the town of Pomfret which is close to the Botswana border (McCulloch, 2002).

(a)

(b)

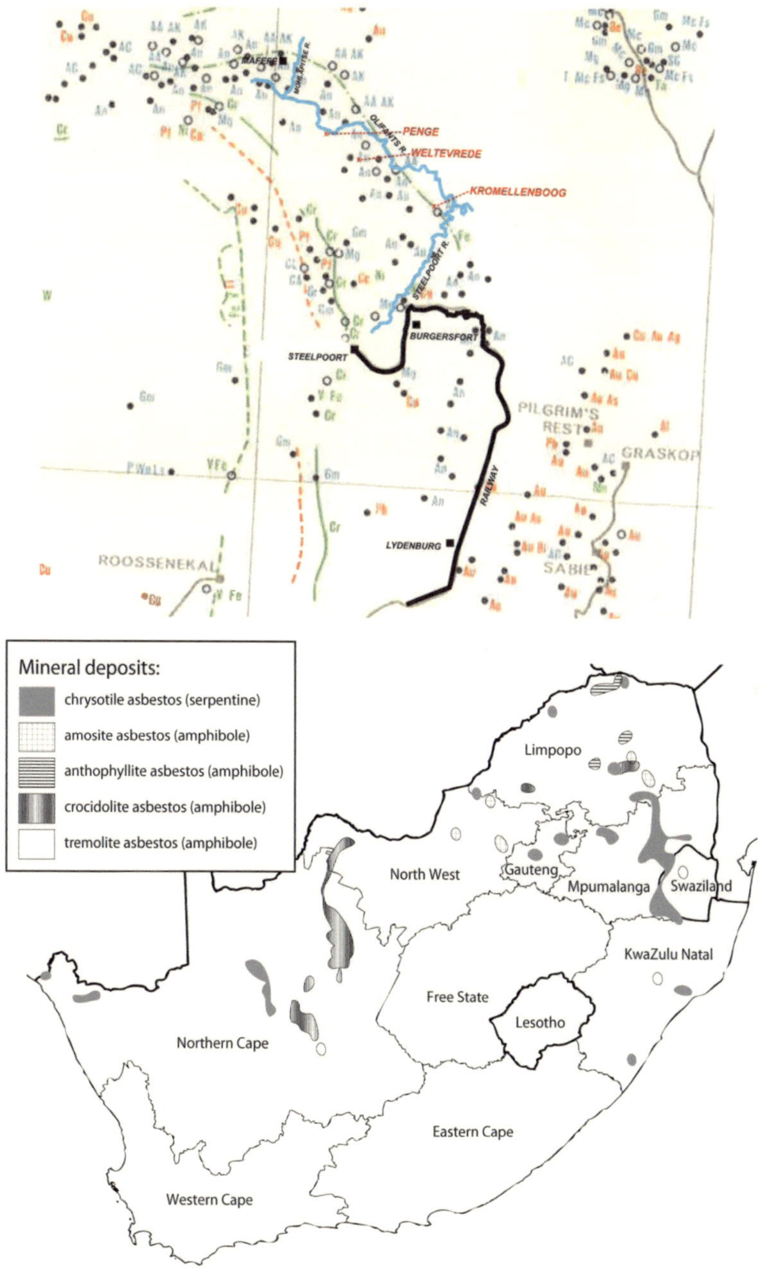

Figure 4. a. Map of the mineral deposits in the Transvaal Crocidolite-Amosite (Pietersburg) asbestos field located on the north-eastern border of the Bushveld Igneous Complex. b. Map of South Africa showing

asbestos deposits. (Courtesy of Dr Gillian Nelson). Key to mineral deposits: AK = Crocidolite, AA = Amosite, AC = Chrysotile, Cr = Chromite, Pt = Platinum, An = Andalusite, Mg = Magnesite, Cu = Copper, V = Vanadium, Pb = Lead, CA = Attapulgite, Ni = Nickel. Modified from: Mineral Map of the Republic of South Africa, an accompaniment to the 1976 publication Mineral Resources of the Republic of South Africa, Department of Mines, Geological Survey, Government Printer, Pretoria ISBN0621034649.

The Pietersburg asbestos field is located in the Limpopo Province along the northern bank of the Olifants River at its western end and on the southern bank from Penge Mine eastwards to Kromellenboog Mine. It terminates on the northern bank of the Steelpoort River just short of its confluence with the Olifants River (29° 30′- 30° 30′E, 24° - 25° S).With the exception of Penge, all the mines are in rugged country and were served by gravel roads until recently. A tarred road links Penge to the railway at Burgersfort. The Pietersburg field is the most complex in geological terms, and seams of amosite and crocidolite are reported to overlap, and the field is sometimes referred to as the Transvaal Crocidolite-Amosite field (Coetzee et al., 1976). It is the source of almost all of the world's supply of amosite and some crocidolite. There is evidence that in the western portion of the field (west of the Mohlapitse River) both crocidolite and amosite are found but that in the eastern part only amosite occurs. In addition to amosite and crocidolite, chrysotile deposits were also mined in the area (Coetzee et al., 1976). The occurrence and exploitation of three asbestos types in the region makes it clear that establishing occupational or environmental exposure to any particular fibre type, and especially to amosite fibre only is not easy or reliable. The only way to determine which fibres an individual has been exposed to is to examine and analyse the fibres retained in the lung and determine the lung fibre burden (Figure 5).

There are numerous deposits of chrysotile in the Mpumalanga, Limpopo and Kwa Zulu Natal Provinces. The most important are in the Barberton area of Mpumalanga where large scale chrysotile mining took place. It was in this region that South Africa's last asbestos mine closed in 2002.

Crocidolite

In South Africa, the first description in the medical literature of malignant mesothelioma of the pleura was the presentation of a single case by Dr Olaf Martiny to the February general meeting of the Transvaal Mine Medical Officers' Association, held at the Witwatersrand Native Labour Association Hospital, in Johannesburg, on the 16th February, 1956 (Martiny, 1956). This case presentation was of a 36 year old Botswana male who was admitted to one of the mine hospitals with pleural thickening and an effusion. Initially he was diagnosed with and treated for tuberculosis. The patient's condition deteriorated and he died. The autopsy and subsequent examination of the tissues was performed by Dr Christopher Wagner who was working at the NIOH (Figure 6). Professor B.J.P. Becker was also present at the autopsy examination. Becker and Wagner's diagnosis was a primary malignant mesothelioma of the pleura. The presentation of this case raised awareness of a hitherto rare pleural tumour presenting with some clinical features that were similar to and initially mistaken for tuberculosis.

Although it is not recorded in the original proceedings of this meeting of the Transvaal Mine Medical Officers Association, Wagner states in his thesis (Wagner, 1962) that in addition to the mesothelioma, histological examination of the lungs showed the presence of asbestosis, asbestos bodies and asbestos fibres. This finding indicates that the patient was significantly exposed to asbestos. Much later, Wagner credits his assistant, Mr D E Munday, with the suggestion to take further sections of the lung which revealed the evidence of asbestos exposure (Wagner, 1991).

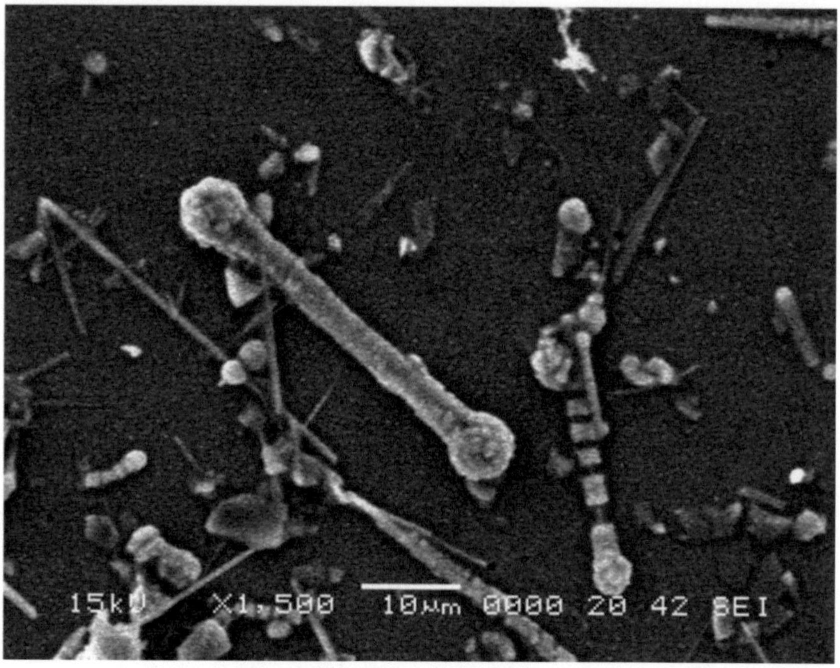

Figure 5. Crocidolite fibres and asbestos bodies from the lung of an asbestos miner. (Courtesy of Professor JI Phillips).

Dr Christopher Sleggs, the medical superintendent of the West End Tuberculosis Hospital, Kimberley, Northern Cape Province, had been concerned about patients with pleural disease who did not respond to the available tuberculosis treatment, and who died. He saw his first patient with what he called atypical tuberculosis in 1952 on a visit to St Konrad's Mission Hospital at Taung and St Michael's Hospital at Bathlaros. He found more cases at Kuruman and began keeping notes on these atypical cases. In 1954, he recorded the histories of two farmers who transported asbestos and were dying of massive pleural tumours. Sleggs observed that patients with pleural tuberculosis coming from areas to the east of Kimberley got better on anti-tuberculosis treatment, but some of those who came from the west, where the crocidolite asbestos fields were, did not respond to treatment and died. Since the early 1950s, Sleggs had referred 12 such patients with clinical features of atypical pleural tuberculosis to thoracic surgeons in Johannesburg, Pretoria, Durban and Cape Town. All were diagnosed as having metastatic carcinomata, not primary mesothelioma of the pleura (McCulloch, 2002).

According to McCulloch, Mr Libero Fatti, the chief thoracic surgical consultant at the Johannesburg General Hospital was called to Kimberley in May 1955 to carry out an emergency operation on an accident victim – a case unrelated to pleural disease. While Fatti was in Kimberley, Sleggs took the opportunity to show him a series of X-rays of what he called atypical tuberculosis. Fatti offered to investigate these cases and arranged for his partner, Mr Paul Marchand, to perform biopsies. Pleural needle biopsies and later open lung biopsies from patients at the West End Hospital were sent to Dr Ian Webster at what is now the NIOH in Johannesburg, who turned them over to his brother in law, Wagner.

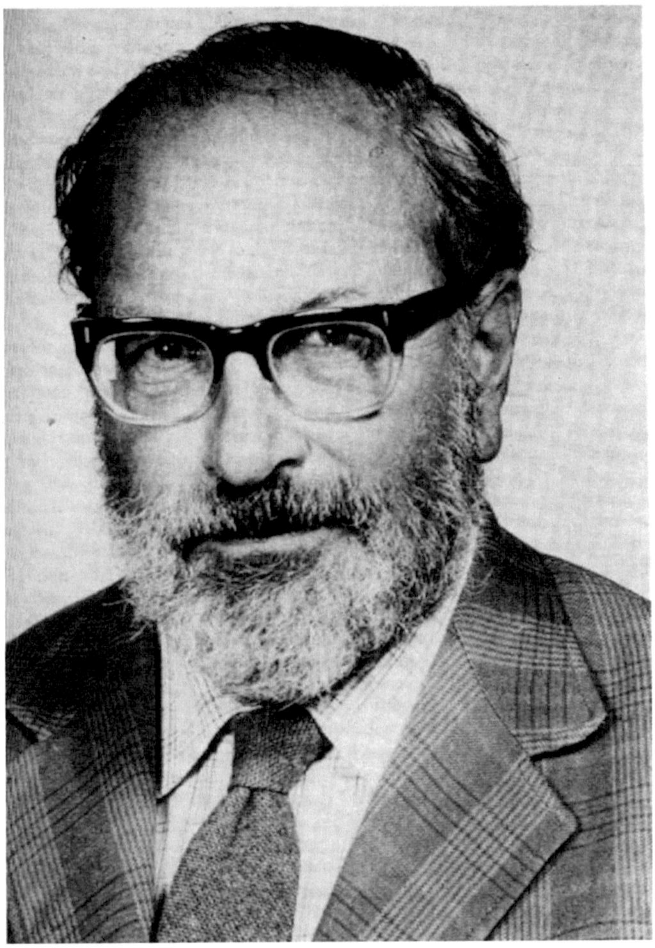

Figure 6. Dr J.C. Wagner. (Courtesy of NIOH archive).

The cases from the West End Hospital formed the basis of the research which led to the publication of two papers (Wagner et al., 1960; Sleggs et al., 1961). The first paper in 1960 reported on 33 cases and the second on 30 of the original cases plus 4 additional cases. By the end of August 1961 Wagner had examined tissue from 78 cases which he collated along with their histories in a table in his thesis (Wagner, 1962). The 1960 paper was to become the most cited paper in the field of occupational health.

All the open lung biopsies from the West End Hospital showed histological features consistent with mesothelioma but it was felt that a definite diagnosis could not be given as "it was not possible to exclude other sites of primary origin"(Wagner, 1962). After examining another 4 cases, the possibility of a common aetiological agent was considered. Because these patients came from the vicinity of the Northern Cape asbestos field, and because evidence of asbestosis and asbestos bodies were seen in the lung tissue of Martiny's case (Martiny, 1956), asbestos exposure was considered by Wagner to be a possible factor. This hypothesis however, could not be supported from the patients' histories, all of whom denied working with asbestos. Their occupations included housewives, domestic servants, cattle herders, farmers, a water bailiff, an assurance agent and an accountant. Subsequently it was discovered that working with asbestos carried a social stigma for all ethnic groups. In addition, many of the patients who had not worked with asbestos did not appreciate the significance of the asbestos mills and dumps in their vicinity (Wagner, 1962).

While the credit for making the association between exposure to asbestos and mesothelioma is generally ascribed to Wagner, several physicians, surgeons and pathologists played a role. The discovery depended on the biopsy material coming to the NIOH, so perhaps, the defining moment was when Sleggs approached Fatti with the X-rays of cases of atypical tuberculosis. The reason for Fatti's presence in Kimberley was serendipitous - he was there for his surgical expertise which was required by an accident victim – not to investigate pleural disease.

A field study, which was conducted by the NIOH in Prieska, Kuruman and Koegas in the Northern Cape from November 1960 to February 1962, concluded that people who were living or who had lived in proximity to asbestos mines or mills were in danger of contracting asbestosis, even though they had no industrial exposure to asbestos dust inhalation. As it was reported: "an alarmingly high number of cases with mesothelioma of the pleura had been discovered among people who have lived in the Northern Cape and that there is evidence that this condition is associated with exposure to asbestos dust inhalation which need not be industrial" (PRU, 1964).

Subsequent studies have shown that almost all cases of mesothelioma in South Africa are associated with exposure to crocidolite asbestos (Webster, 1973; Cochrane and Webster, 1978; Rees et al., 1999a; Nolan et al., 2006). Webster considered the association with mesothelioma to be a peculiar property of Cape crocidolite (Webster, 1973). In a study of 7317 white male employees in amosite and crocidolite mines, excluding miners of Transvaal crocidolite, it was shown that crocidolite miners were approximately 7 times more likely to develop mesothelioma than amosite miners (Sluis-Cremer et al., 1992).

A case control study of 123 South African cases of mesothelioma showed a preponderance of cases where the exposure was attributed to crocidolite (Rees et al., 1999a). In this study, 5 of the patients had no known history of exposure to asbestos. Of the remainder, 82% were occupationally exposed and 18% environmentally exposed. Of the environmentally exposed patients, 91% had contact with Cape crocidolite. There was a relative paucity of cases linked to amosite and none of the cases could be linked convincingly to chrysotile exposure. The conclusion of this study is that there is a fibre gradient of mesotheliomagenic potential for South African asbestos. The mesotheliomagenic potential for crocidolite is greater than that for amosite which is greater than that for chrysotile.

In an attempt to produce a definitive study of fibre type in cases of histologically proven mesothelioma, inorganic material was recovered from the lung parenchyma of 43 South African cases of mesothelioma. Using analytical transmission electron microscopy the types and concentrations of fibrous minerals were determined. Crocidolite was found to be the most frequently occurring fibre type. In 7 of the 9 cases with more than a million fibres per gram of dried lung tissue, at least 85% of the fibres were crocidolite. Crocidolite occurred alone in 12 of the 33 occupationally exposed cases and in 3 of the 4 environmentally exposed cases. In the fourth environmental case, 96% of the fibres were crocidolite. When the total asbestos concentration in the lung was less than 250,000 fibres per gram of dried lung tissue, crocidolite was the only fibre type identified. The mean concentration of crocidolite for all 43 cases was 270,000 fibres per gram of dried lung tissue. This fibre burden is substantially below the lung burden of chrysotile fibres in general populations without asbestos-related disease (Langer et al., 1971; Langer and Nolan, 1994). This study supports the hypothesis that mesothelioma can develop in individuals following exposures to crocidolite that may be brief or slight (Nolan et al., 2006).

Some types of mining work carried a high risk for developing mesothelioma; an example of this would be cobbing. Crocidolite and amosite occur in banded ironstone which is extremely hard. Cobbers removed adherent ironstone from the ends of cobs of fibre with a hammer in order to prevent the mills breaking down from the impact of the ironstone. They would work sitting all day long hammering at asbestos bearing rock less than half a metre from their breathing zone. A group of 53 women cobbers of crocidolite were examined at St Michael's Mission Hospital in the Northern Cape Province. Twelve of these 53 cobbers developed mesothelioma (Talent et al., 1978).

The mining of Transvaal crocidolite in the Pietersburg field came to an end in 1976 and the mining of crocidolite in the Northern Cape ceased in 1996. During the time the mines were active, exposure levels to asbestos fibres were high (McCulloch, 2002). Records of exposure levels are poor and sparse. A dust survey at the Dublin Consolidated blending plant in Pietersburg found an average concentration of 179 fibres/ml in 1966 and 40 fibres/ml in 1974. At eight small mines in the Limpopo Province around Mafefe the fibre levels varied from 1 to 89 fibres/ml (Felix, 1997).

Studies on data collected on mesothelioma occurring in specific geographical areas of South Africa showed high rates of mesothelioma in areas where Cape crocidolite was mined. A study conducted in five Cape crocidolite-mining magisterial districts was based on death registrations from 1968 to 1980 (Botha et al., 1986). The authors calculated standardised mortality ratios (SMRs) for asbestosis and/or mesothelioma, without distinguishing between the two diseases. Rates, compared to the control group, were significantly elevated for men and women of all races, with SMRs of 7.86 for white men, 10.3 for white women, and 8.43 and 8.72 for men and women of mixed race, respectively.

A birth cohort was established in one of the magisterial districts in which the above study was conducted (Reid et al., 1990; Kielkowski et al., 2000). The cohort comprised men and women whose births were registered from 1916 to 1936. By 1995, 74% of white men and women had been traced compared to 13 to 22% of other race groups. Analysis was thus restricted to white cohort members. The crude mortality rates for mesothelioma were 366 and 172 per million person-years for men and women, respectively.

The evidence from studies of South African cases of mesothelioma is consistent in showing that the dominant fibre type responsible is Cape crocidolite. The data for Transvaal crocidolite is sparse. The Transvaal crocidolite mines were smaller operations and were often excluded from studies, or pooled with amosite mines (Sluis-Cremer et al., 1992; Rees et al., 1999a; Rees et al., 1999b). Part of the legacy of South Africa's exploitation of its asbestos mineral reserves is the large number of cases of mesothelioma caused by environmental exposure. These environmentally exposed cases, in particular, appear to be the result of exposure to crocidolite.

Amosite

An important feature of the South African experience in respect of malignant mesothelioma is the prominence of environmental exposure. This has been identified since the very first published paper (Wagner, 1960) on the association of blue fibre and malignant mesothelioma. The section on amosite makes it clear at the outset that determining exposure to a specific fibre only in the Pietersburg field is difficult. This is clear from detailed mapping, from west to east, of the geological transition from a succession of crocidolite and amosite seams at Malips River, to the dominance of amosite at the Mohlapitse River, to amosite only at Penge mine (Figures 7 and 8) and at Kromellenboog mine (Coetzee, 1976).

The vast majority of occupational medicine studies are carried out and published without environmental measurements. In this respect the Pietersburg field is unusual as there are reliable measurements of both occupational and environmental exposure. The two studies summarized in this chapter are unique in their attention to detail and the spread of the findings. This account seeks to add new data to the inconclusive situation in the Pietersburg field and the studies of amosite miners, as opposed to insulators and laggers.

The health effects of amosite mining and milling in South Africa have been reviewed in detail (Murray and Nelson, 2008). There is sound evidence of occupational and environmental exposure to airborne amosite fibre in the Pietersburg asbestos field for more than fifty years. In her thesis, Felix cites the early description of 'unchecked' exposures of children at work in the mill at Penge Mine. It was then one of the largest asbestos mines in the world and the source of most of the supply of amosite. Schepers, an officer of the Medical Bureau for Occupational Diseases in Johannesburg, visited Penge Mine in 1949 and commented thus: "Exposures were crude and unchecked. I found children, completely included within large shipping bags, trampling down fluffy amosite asbestos, which all day came cascading down over their heads"(Felix, 1997).

Labour was drawn, in the main, from the rural areas surrounding the mines (Davies et al., 2004). The Penge group of mines (Penge, Weltevrede and Kromellenboog) operated a recruiting depot in the Eastern Cape, in what was formerly the Transkei, which was used to recruit additional labour when labour shortages occurred locally.

Rendall, working at the National Institute for Occupational Health, carried out a detailed survey of Penge mine in 1970 (Rendall and Davies, 2007). He collected 267 full-shift personal samples from underground and surface workers at Penge mine in 1971-72. The average of 94 personal samples collected from individuals working underground was 1.34 fibres(f)/ml (range 0.28-3.26) The median value for the individuals grouped by task or work station and averaged (22 groups) was 1.10 f/ml. This low level and narrow range of exposure is attributed to the fact that the underground workings at Penge mine are kept constantly wet by water dripping from the hanging walls and running down the side walls, acting as a dust suppressant. The ore leaving the underground workings is saturated. In stark contrast the average of 177 personal samples collected from individuals working above ground in the offices, workshops, mills and packing departments, where the material being processed is dry, was 25 f/ml (range 0.28-326.7). The median value for the individuals grouped by task or work station and averaged (24 groups) was 37.2 f/ml. The highest fibre level was associated with hand tamping in the packing process – exactly the situation described by Schepers (see Felix 1997) except for the fact that there were no children jumping up and down in the bags. Rendall also measured the total dust levels and calculated the number of fibres per milligram of dust, showing that the total dust level did not correlate well with the fibre exposure. In the assay laboratory the total dust level was 2.68 mg/m^3 containing 24.1 million fibres/mg whereas in quality control the dust level of 0.55 mg/m^3 contained 21.3 million f/mg. and in the bagging plant 21 million fibres. This illustrates the importance of the relationship between the process and the fibre content of the dust.

Simultaneously Cape Asbestos, the owners of Penge, operated a smaller mine or set of mines known as Egnep at Malipsdrift towards the western extremity of the Pietersburg field 60 kilometres west of Penge Mine. Officially Penge and Egnep were considered as one mine, and the product from these mines, well to the west of the Mohlapitse River, was transported to Penge for shipment via the railway siding at Apiesdoring near Burgersfort.

The association of the mining operation at Malipsdrift with that at Penge and the uncertainty as to where deposits of Transvaal crocidolite end and pure amosite begins implies a possibility, if not of admixture in the product, at least of mixed exposure of workers. Production of amosite from Penge and the smaller mines along the northern bank of the Olifants River peaked in 1970 at 100,000 tonnes. At that stage 7,000 men were employed at Penge. Cape Asbestos had major crocidolite mining operations in the Northern Cape, and senior employees were interchanged or made visits to Cape's other mines. This adds a further complication to the accurate determination of exclusive fibre type exposure. Some experienced foremen were also moved from the crocidolite to the amosite mines and vice versa.

Environmental exposure was investigated in detail as part of the study of the villages round Mafefe. The results are recorded here to make the point that one would expect a significant number of environment only cases from Mafefe and the many similar groups of villages situated in close proximity to asbestos mines in the Pietersburg field. In 1990, as part of the study cited previously, Felix investigated the "current sources of environmental asbestos exposure in Mafefe" where a number of small mines worked deposits of amosite and

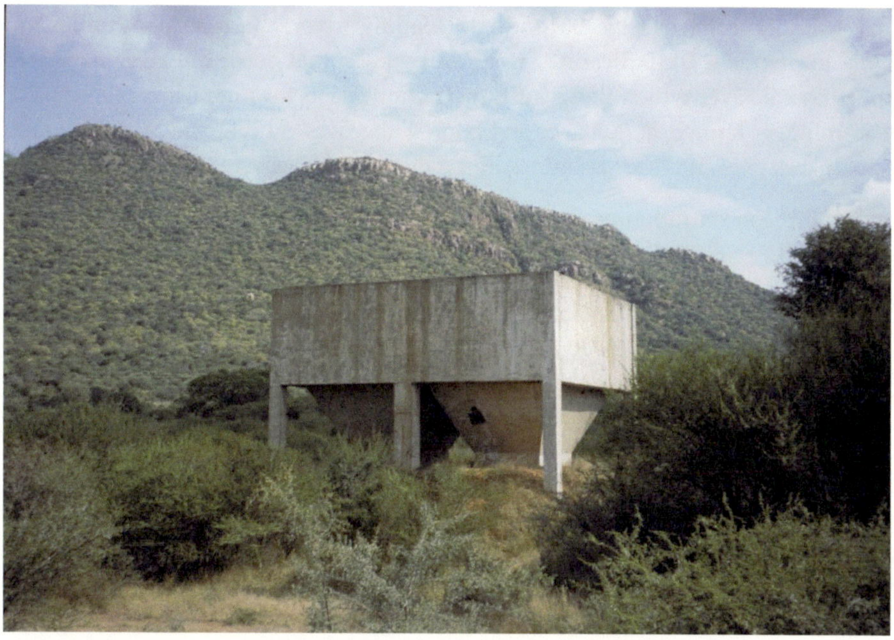

Figure 7. Derelict ore bins at Penge mine. (Courtesy of Dr Koichi Honma).

crocidolite, via surface workings, adits or less often from underground workings (Figure 8). Their tailings dumps were close to one or more of the 30 settlements which fall under the jurisdiction of the traditional ruler (kgosi) in the Mafefe area. The population of Mafefe in November 1987 was 11,119. Tailings were frequently dumped on the banks of the Mohlapitse River or the streams draining into it. Deposits high in the Strydpoort Mountains were worked from adits and the waste rock and tailings tipped down the hillside – to this day the resulting environmental contamination cannot be abated in this rugged terrain. This doctoral thesis is a rich source of historical and contemporary information, and includes detailed maps and lists of fibre levels measured by government inspectors over the years – it would be instructive to reproduce more of the detail in the thesis but this would make the account unwieldy. Thorough investigations of asbestos exposure in communities living around asbestos mines, such as this one, are rare.

Ninety-two personal samples were collected by adults and children going about their usual tasks. The mean of the 92 samples was 12 fibres per litre or 12,000 f/m^3 (0.6 – 90 f/l; S.D. 13.3 f/l). Fourteen samples showed levels above 20 f/l. The highest mean concentration of fibres was 20.3 f/l among children playing (13 samples). School attendance exposed children to a mean of 13.2 f/l (9 samples), and teachers were exposed to 12.5 f/l (5 samples). Usual activities such as building and gardening entailed exposure to 16.1f/l (8 samples) and 15 f/l (7 samples) respectively. Walking about the village exposed subjects to 12.0 f/l (9 samples) and housework entailed exposure to 8.6 f/l (16 samples).

The tailings dumps on the bank of streams feeding the Mohlapitse River have been mentioned. The seasonally dry bed of this river is used as a source of building sand. Two personal samples collected by individuals loading river sand onto a trailer revealed exposures to 4 and 12 f/l, indicating significant contamination of the river bed. This river joins the Olifants River which flows into the Indian Ocean through Mozambique. Needless to say nothing is known about asbestos-related diseases among the riparian population living downstream of the asbestos mines in the Pietersburg asbestos field.

The mean fibre concentration of 62 strategic samples was 11 f/l or 11,000 f/m^3 (range 0.1 – 51.2 f/l; S.D.11.7 f/l). Two results were excluded; one taken alongside a children's playground (756.5 f/l) and another (50.4 f/l) taken inside a house in which there was no visible asbestos in the construction. These levels were judged to be aberrant and no explanation could be found. The mean of 44 outdoor strategic samples was 14.5 f/l (s.d. 13.9), and that of 18 taken indoors was 2.7 f/l (s.d. 1.8). On days when vehicles used the road, the mean of 12 strategic samples taken at the roadside was 20.7 f/l (s.d. 14.8) compared with 13.1 f/l (s.d. 14.5) on the 10 vehicle free days.

Finally, the extent and variability of environmental asbestos exposure is clearly established by two series of strategic measurements made in 7 villages in close proximity (less than 1 kilometre) to tailings dumps and 11 villages far (more than 1.5 kilometre) from dumps. The mean fibre concentration in ambient air collected by strategic sampling in villages close to the dumps (21 samples) was 18.6 f/l, and in the rest (23 samples) 10.8f/l. The difference is statistically significant ($p < 0.00001$). The unofficial limit for environmental exposure was set at 20 f/l. It is reasonable to conclude that residents of Mafefe were exposed intermittently to levels higher than this, and regularly to lowerlevels.

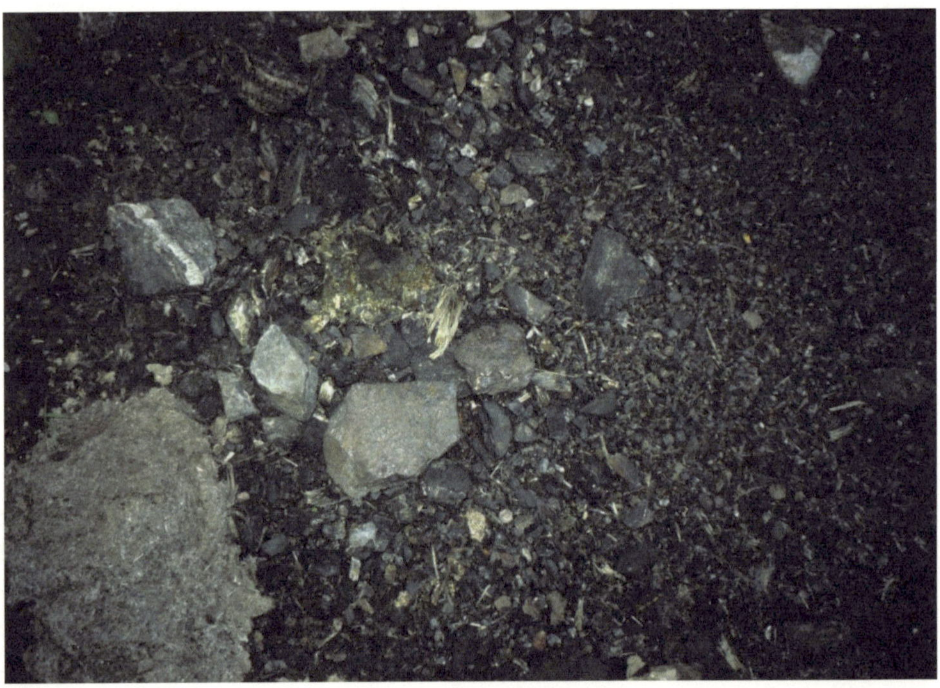

Figure 8. Amosite fibres contaminating the ground near Penge mine. (Courtesy of Dr Koichi Honma).

Given this degree of occupational and environmental exposure of the labour force, and the communities from which they were drawn, one might be justified in assuming that a situation comparable to that described in the study of the crocidolite-exposed Prieska birth cohort might be found in the area. This is not the case.

Felix (Felix, 1997) analysed the available data from two studies of autopsy findings in cardio-respiratory organs submitted from Penge Mine and from mines in the Northern Cape (Sluis-Cremer, 1965, 1970). The figures presented show a higher prevalence of asbestosis at Penge and, in addition, a much smaller improvement over time at Penge. The numbers of autopsies analysed, the age and length of service of the two groups do not differ significantly. There is a significant body of evidence of widespread benign pleural and parenchymal asbestos related respiratory disease among occupationally and environmentally exposed individuals. There are sporadic, unconfirmed reports of mesotheliomas.

In a random sample of 892 adults from a census of Mafefe, where a number of small mines worked deposits of amosite and crocidolite, 681 were examined. Pleural changes which could be confidently classified as asbestos-related pleural disease were present in 35% of women and 52% of men, with a significant upward trend with age (Felix, 1997).

In terms of the Occupational Diseases in Mines and Works Act 1973, doctors in South Africa are required to report occupational lung disease in current or former mine workers to the Medical Bureau for Occupational Diseases (MBOD) in Johannesburg. Reports from doctors working in the hospitals and clinics in and around the Pietersburg asbestos field were very uncommon prior to 1991. When a clinic was established at Groothoek Hospital to service the need for compensation examinations at Mafefe, no reports had ever been received from that hospital by the MBOD. Sustained attempts were made from November 1991 onwards to interview and examine former asbestos miners for compensation purposes, with the assistance of local activists. In the period 1991-1994, reports for 927 former asbestos miners were submitted to the MBOD. During an intensive case finding project in 1996 more than 2000 former miners were examined and reported (Davies et al., 2001). A number of publications resulted and these show a high prevalence of benign asbestos-related diseases, but did not identify any substantial number of proven malignant mesotheliomas or lung cancers (Davies et al., 2001; Davies et al., 2004).

The first report of a malignant mesothelioma from the area of the Pietersburg asbestos field, which has overlapping seams of amosite and crocidolite fibres, is contained in a review of 485 females and 53 males admitted to the medical wards of the Jane Furse Memorial Mission Hospital situated about 60 kilometres south-west of Penge Mine (Edginton et al., 1972). At the time the hospital was estimated to be responsible for the medical care of 100,000 people. Forty-eight per cent (231) of the diagnoses in women were respiratory disease - tuberculosis 98, other respiratory infections 130. Non-infective respiratory disorders were found in only three women – one autopsy proven malignant pleural mesothelioma, and one possible but unproven lung cancer, and one case of asthma. Despite the proximity of asbestos mining, asbestos-related disease is not mentioned in the discussion. The high incidence of respiratory disease and a single mesothelioma in a series of fewer than 500 female patients is surely remarkable, and worthy of comment. However, we have no information about these patients' occupation or exposure history.

Further unverified evidence of mesotheliomas from the Pietersburg field is included in the Felix thesis. Felix's personal communication in 1990 with Dr van Rensburg, a pathologist working at the Pietersburg laboratory of the South African Institute for Medical Research (SAIMR) reads: "In 15 months from February 1989 to April 1990, 16 mesothliomas were diagnosed at the SAIMR Pietersburg laboratory. Of the 16 cases, 11 occurred in black persons, 4 of whom were women". No details of occupation or exposure are given.

In 1990 a 44 year old migrant worker who worked for 2 years from 1963 to 1965 on an asbestos mine in the Pietersburg asbestos field, was diagnosed as having a mesothelioma at the Rand Mutual Hospital, Johannesburg (Felix, 1997). No details of the mine on which he was employed are available.

Serious reservations must be clearly stated before an attempt is made to make any conclusive statement about the relationship between occupational and/or environmental amosite exposure and the occurrence of malignant mesothelial tumours. The first proviso is that related to the overlapping fibre types in the Pietersburg field. Additional reservations include the inaccessible area in which amosite was mined, the rudimentary medical services in the area surrounding the amosite mines and the apparent neglect by the mine itself, all of which hamper us in getting conclusive data about amosite exposure.

In the dust rooms of the National Centre for Occupational Health non-human primates were exposed to specific dusts, including amosite, and kept in the laboratory for many years in order to determine the long term effects of the dusts to which they had been exposed. The non-human primates used in the experiments were locally captured baboons (*Papio ursinus*). At the time, there was no evidence that South African baboons were natural hosts for SV40 (Malherbe, 1974). In one study, 12 baboons were exposed to amosite for a period of between 242 days and 898 days. Exposures were high, ranging between 1100 and 1200 fibres per cc. Ten survived the exposure period and lived for a further 1.2 to 10.2 years. Five of these 10 baboons developed mesothelioma: 3 were peritoneal and 2 were pleural tumours (Webster et al., 1993). The amosite used in these exposure studies was the milled sample prepared at the NIOH for the UICC standard reference sample. This amosite standard reference sample has been used in asbestos-exposure related research studies worldwide (Timbrell and Rendall, 1971; Rendall, 1980). It is possible that the milling of the fibre may alter its physical properties thereby increasing its toxicity, in contrast to the freshly mined fibres. This may provide another possible explanation for the apparent rarity of malignant mesotheliomas among miners exposed to freshly mined amosite fibre.

Rees debates the role of amosite in the causation of malignant mesothelioma in the course of a case-control study of 123 cases and 119 cancer controls and 103 medical controls. The conclusion is carefully stated and is quoted in full: "The relative importance of Cape crocidolite should not mask the impact of identifying three cases in 16 months from a single amosite mine (Penge). This, together with the contention by Felix (Felix et al., 1994) that mesothelioma is under-diagnosed in the North Eastern Transvaal (now Limpopo and Mpumalanga Provinces), provides motivation for case-finding strategies in the area. Cross-sectional surveys are inappropriate for a rare disease with short life expectancy following diagnosis, so alternatives are necessary. One approach would be to allocate the task to the regional health authority which would be in a position to identify cases by encouraging pathologists to submit suspect tissue for expert review. Cases could be identified by establishing diagnostic and compensation services for asbestos-related diseases in the major regional hospital and by providing information about the condition and the service to the community and local medical practitioners"(Rees et al., 1999b).

Since this was written many thousands of former asbestos workers have been examined for compensation purposes in the Pietersburg asbestos field (Davies et al., 2001; Davies et al., 2004). The Maandagshoek Project set up a network of clinics in co-operation with a number of community-based activists following five years of preliminary work at Groothoek Hospital. Workers who had been certified by the MBOD were subsequently denied compensation by an administrative decision making written records of mining employment obligatory. In an interesting report South Africa's Public Protector declared this to be unconstitutional and stated that there were 12,000 outstanding claims which should be reviewed (Public-Protector, 2008). Among the thousands of applicants for benefits interviewed and examined as part of the Maandagshoek Project there were no proven mesotheliomas.

The study of asbestos fibre type and mesothelioma carried out on cases autopsied at the NIOH demonstrates a residual burden of exclusively amosite fibres in only one of 43 cases examined. In five cases amosite was the majority fibre type (more than 50%) accompanied in all cases by crocidolite in proportions ranging from 7-33%. In six cases amosite was the second most common fibre (4-22%), crocidolite being the dominant fibre in each of these. The remainder of the cases were attributable to crocidolite (Nolan R P, 2006).

Occupational and environmental exposures to asbestos in the Pietersburg field were high and high rates of benign asbestos-related disease have been described (Murray and Nelson, 2008). But mesothelioma is rarely reported from the hospitals and clinics in and around the Pietersburg asbestos field. The reporting of asbestos-related disease is extremely poor in South Africa, particularly in the areas that supplied labour to the mines (Talent et al., 1978). There is an underlying problem in attributing cases of mesothelioma to amosite because of the geological relationship between deposits of amosite and Transvaal crocidolite. The single case from the Jane Furse Hospital and the unconfirmed series of cases reported from the SAIMR laboratory in Pietersburg have no occupational histories or exposure data. The nearest we have to definitive studies are the doctoral thesis by Rees (Rees, 1995) and the residual fibre study by Nolan (Nolan, 2006). Both of these suggest that amosite plays a minor role and that crocidolite is much more important. By comparison with the Northern Cape, where crocidolite is mined, environmental mesotheliomas in proximity to amosite mines and mills are rare.

Chrysotile

The role of chrysotile in the causation of mesothelioma has been debated for decades (Churg, 1988; Huncharek, 1994; Smith and Wright, 1996; Stayner et al., 1996; Egilman et al., 2003; McDonald, 2010). One view is that the amphiboles (crocidolite, amosite and tremolite) explain almost all cases of mesothelioma and that "chrysotile mesothelioma" is induced by contaminating tremolite (McDonald, 2010). A contrasting opinion is that chrysotile is the main cause of mesothelioma (Smith and Wright, 1996). The South African experience of mesothelioma and chrysotile is of interest in this debate because the country mined, milled, transported and used large quantities of the fibre.

Chrysotile mining started in South Africa in about 1920 (Felix et al., 1994). From 1975 to 1992 production was close to 100 000 US tons per annum. From 1992 output declined dramatically to about 20 000 tons in 2000 (Rees et al., 2001). The mining of chrysotile asbestos ceased when the last mine at Msauli closed in 2002. Exports of chrysotile overtook that of amosite in the mid-1970s and crocidolite in the early 1980s (Harington and McGlashan, 1998). From 1980 to 2003, 1,568,928 metric tonnes of chrysotile had been exported, making up 54% of South Africa's total asbestos export over the period (Harington et al., 2010). Substantial numbers of miners produced the mineral: from the 1930s to mid-1980s roughly 1000- 2000 miners were employed at any time with a peak of about 2 600 in 1960 - 17% of all asbestos miners in that year (Rees et al., 1999a).

In South Africa, despite the substantial output and large numbers exposed, mesothelioma attributable to exposure to chrysotile-only has not been convincingly documented. The first paper to comment on this issue was published by Webster in 1973 (Webster, 1973), who reviewed the exposure histories of 232 cases of pleural mesothelioma referred to South Africa's Asbestos Tumour Reference Panel. Seventy eight of the cases had been exposed during mining operations, 75 of them (96%) on crocidolite mines and three (4%) on Penge amosite mine. Webster reported that there were no cases in which there had been exposure to chrysotile only, but noted that relatively small numbers of miners were employed in chrysotile mining. Five years later, the exposure histories of 70 additional cases were published (Cochrane and Webster, 1978). Fibre-specific exposures were not reported except for 13 cases with non-occupational environmental exposure associated with mining: all 13 of them had been exposed in the Northern Cape crocidolite fields. In 1984, Solomons published a review of 80 cases of mesothelioma referred to the occupational medicine clinic of the NIOH, during 1977 to 1983 (Solomons, 1984). Fibre type was thought to be mixed in most cases. Documented exposure in 17 cases was to Cape crocidolite only and in four cases to amosite only (Penge mine). Although not explicitly stated, it can be assumed that no chrysotile-only case was found in this study.

In 1986, Wagner supported the view that mesothelioma was rare or non-existent in South African chrysotile miners by stating that the malignancy had not been recorded among these workers (Wagner, 1986). Surprisingly little research was conducted subsequently on mesothelioma in relation to this fibre type, but in 1999 the exposure histories of 123 consecutive incident cases diagnosed or treated in six South African cities were published (Rees et al., 1999a; Rees et al., 1999b). The cases were interviewed in life and details of domestic, environmental and occupational asbestos exposure were obtained. No case had a history of chrysotile mining or environmental contact exclusively with this fibre type. Two cases (1.6%) reported contact with chrysotile and little if any contact with amphiboles, but neither was conclusive of chrysotile as the cause of the mesothelioma. One had been exposed to the mineral only four years prior to diagnosis. The other had spent over 30 years in chrysotile mining districts but had spent three months on an asbestos mine in the Northern Province - an amphibole mining area. In a biopsy of his pleural tissue, amphibole asbestos fibres were isolated (Rees et al., 1999a).

The most recent data are from two trusts which were established in 2003 and 2006 following litigation by claimants seeking compensation for asbestos-related diseases. The trusts are respectively the Asbestos Relief Trust (ART) and the Kgalagadi Relief Trust (KRT)(KRT, 2011). The ART provides for those exposed at or near 30 asbestos mines and related operations including all of the major chrysotile mines. The KRT provides only for claimants with exposure arising from two crocidolite mines. To date 275 cases of mesothelioma have been adjudicated, none from a chrysotile area (Mothemela, 2011). Additional information comes from the personal experience of pathologists at the NIOH. The NIOH Pathology Division conducts autopsies on former miners to ascertain eligibility for workers' compensation. All deceased miners are entitled to an autopsy. According to the Head of Pathology, no case of a mesothelioma has been recorded in a miner with service only in chrysotile mining (Personal communication Murray J, NIOH 2011). This is despite fairly large numbers of former miners with mesothelioma coming to autopsy: 111 cases from 2004 to 2007 (Phillips and Murray, 2009).

There are a number of possible explanations for the absence or paucity of documented chrysotile mesothelioma cases in South Africa. First, this may be a consequence of very small numbers of people having had exposure to chrysotile fibre. This explanation is unconvincing given the fairly large numbers employed in the industry over many decades. Second, it may well be that these cases are rare and have been missed. Based on cohort studies of workers predominantly exposed to chrysotile, it has been estimated that overall about 0.3% of these workers died of mesothelioma, although the percentage of deaths varied across the exposure settings and was influenced by time passed since first exposure and ascertainment of cohort vital status and cause of death (Stayner et al., 1996). Even at peak employment in South African chrysotile mining - 2 600 people – there would have been 7.8 mesothelioma cases in this cohort at an estimated risk of 0.3%. Thus, despite over 80 years of chrysotile mining, the number of cases may be relatively small, but it seems unlikely that all of them would have been unrecorded. A third explanation is that exposure was so well controlled that cases would not arise. Again, this is unlikely. Slade, a medical officer at a chrysotile mine, observed in 1931 that: "Several years of experience at the mill has shown that the concentration of dust in the atmosphere in that building is at all times excessive, and frequently sufficiently so [as] to render indistinguishable objects at a distance of a few yards." (Felix et al., 1994).

It should be noted, though, that management of African Chrysotile Asbestos (ACA), by far the largest chrysotile mine, has stated that fibre levels were consistently below 1 fibre/ml in the 1980s and 90s (Rees et al., 2001). These measurements were not independently verified and the statement may have been based on average fibre concentrations, rather than the exposure levels of the most exposed miners and millers (Rees et al., 2001). Given the low credibility of the former explanations for the paucity of mesotheliomas attributable to chrysotile-only exposure, a relatively low level of contamination of South African chrysotile by tremolite deserves consideration. Unfortunately, data on this issue are scanty: only two small studies have been published (Rees et al., 1992; Rees et al., 2001). Additionally, there has been one small unpublished dust survey done by the NIOH (du Toit, 1992). In the first study, tremolite fibres were sought in the lungs of four subjects with service exceeding 20 years on chrysotile mines. Scanning electron microscopy demonstrated tremolite in two of the four, but the fibres were scanty: one fibre seen in about 20 fields at 1000 times magnification. In the second study, asbestos fibre concentrations were determined in the lungs of nine South African chrysotile mine workers. Despite long service in most (range: unknown - 32 years; median, 9 years), asbestos fibre concentrations were generally low (geometric mean 690,000 and 330,000 fibres/gram dried lung tissue for chrysotile and tremolite respectively). The tremolite:chrysotile ratio was greater than one in only a single case. Both these findings are in contrast to those observed for Canadian chrysotile miners who have been shown to have much higher lung fibre burdens and a general preponderance of tremolite over chrysotile (Becklake and Case, 1994; Churg, 1994; Rees et al., 2001). The unpublished study (du Toit, 1992) examined 20 rock samples, two bulk dust samples from the mill and seven samples of airborne dust from ACA mine. Tremolite was found in only one rock sample; the dust samples were inconclusive (possible tremolite); and one tremolite fibre was identified in each of two of the seven air samples. Taken together, these three pieces of information, although far from conclusive, are suggestive of relatively low tremolite contamination and offer a plausible explanation for the lack of mesotheliomas in South Africa attributable to chrysotile exposure alone.

2. Non-occupational mesothelioma in South Africa

South Africa has a uniquely high national burden of environmental mesothelioma (i.e. cases with only non-occupational asbestos exposure). Environmental mesothelioma and the role of fibre type has been reviewed (White et al., 2008). Table 1 shows a consistently high proportion of these cases – 8.8% to 33% - from a variety of South African studies.

The lowest proportion was derived from a series of cases referred to an occupational medicine clinic (Solomons, 1984), and the intention to claim workers' compensation for an occupational disease probably led to a referral bias of subjects exposed at work. At that time, occupationally-induced cases were compensable but not those that were environmentally-induced. The highest proportion of environmentally induced mesotheliomas (33%) was from a study of cases registered with the South African Asbestos Tumour Reference Panel (Webster, 1973). Exposure histories were obtained from an interview with the patient (percentage not stated) or from a proforma completed by the medical practitioner submitting the biopsy specimen. Exposure histories were missing in 9% and no asbestos exposure was recorded for a further 14%. It is likely that thorough interrogation for

Reference	Source of mesothelioma subjects	Proportion environmental	Definition of environmental	Comment
(Webster, 1973)	232 cases registered with the South African Asbestos Tumour Reference Panel, 1955-1970	33%	No occupational exposure	Exposure histories usually taken by submitting doctor
(Cochrane and Webster, 1978)	70 cases referred to the National Research Institute for Occupational Disease, Johannesburg, by local practitioners	18.6%	Minimum 3 years residence in a mining area with no occupational exposure	Exposure history taken by authors from patients in-life
(Solomons, 1984)	80 cases referred to National Centre for Occupational Health clinic, Johannesburg, 1977 to 1983	8.8%	No occupational exposure	Exposure histories taken by clinic doctors from patients. Referral to the clinic probably influenced by intention to claim workers' compensation
(Zwi et al., 1989)	1347 cases identified by South African practitioners, 1976-1984	Males: 10% Females: 35% Total: 16%	Lived in the north-western Cape asbestos belt, or had specified domestic exposure with no occupational exposure	Exposure data supplied by reporting practitioner. No information available on 33% of cases
(Rees et al., 1999a)	123 cases diagnosed or treated in 6 South African cities, late 1988-early 1990	17.9%	Spent time in asbestos mining area without occupational exposure. Two cases also lived or worked in asbestos cement structures	Detailed exposure history taken in-life from cases
(Kielkowski et al., 2000)	28 cases from a birth cohort of white South Africans born in Prieska district (a crocidolite mining area) 1916-1936	Estimated 29%	All women cases (8/28) considered environmental	No exposure data but white women rarely worked in asbestos industries
(White et al., 2008)	Review of 504 cases	23% in total	Histologically proven cases	Exposure data for 87% of cases
(Mothemela, 2011)	295 compensation claimants adjudicated by ART and KRT*, 2003-2010	29.2%	Claimant must have resided within 10 kms of a qualifying operation (e.g. mine or mill) without occupational asbestos contact	Exposure histories obtained from claimants files. Trusts provided compensation for environmental and occupational exposure

*ART = Asbestos Relief Trust; KRT = Kgalagadi Relief Trust.

Table 1. Proportions of South African mesothelioma cases considered to be environmental

occupational exposure was inconsistent as workers' compensation for mesothelioma was only provided for miners from 1962 and for non-mining workers from 1979 (Solomons, 1984), whereas the cases were collected from 1955-1970. The Kielkowski study (Kielkowski et al., 2000) did not have exposure data, but assumed environmental exposure in all women subjects; if even a small proportion had had occupational exposure the 29% proportion would be reduced. The Mothemela data (Mothemela, 2011) are not generalisable to the country as a whole as these data are from claimants who either lived near or worked at mining operations. The other studies also have methodological limitations, e.g. 33% of the subjects in the Zwi study did not have exposure histories (Zwi et al., 1989). In a review of 504 cases from four of the above studies (White et al., 2008), the exposure was attributed to the environment in 23% in total. The 1973 Webster and 1984 Solomons studies are probably the least reliable in terms of proportions of environmentally-induced cases; if these two are ignored the remaining studies are fairly consistent: in South African mining regions the proportion of environmental cases is in the order of 29% (Kielkowski et al., 2000; Mothemela, 2011) and between 16% and 19% for the country as a whole (Zwi et al., 1989; Rees et al., 1999a; Cochrane and Webster, 1978).

This high environmental burden is in sharp contrast to other settings, except for the Wittenoom crocidolite mining region of northwest Australia; Da-yao, southwestern China, a region with naturally scattered patches of crocidolite ore; and central Anatolia in Turkey, where soil is contaminated with tremolite or tremolite-actinolite-chrysotile mixtures and less so with anthophyllite-chrysotile mixtures. During 1979-1994, 176 Wittenoom mesothelioma cases were documented of whom 34 (19.3%) had not been employed in mining, milling or transport of asbestos, but had lived in or visited the area (Rogers and Nevill, 1995). The 34 cases arose over 16 years; about two non-occupational cases per year. The population of three villages of Da-yao with about 20% of the total ground surface covered by crocidolite ore has been about 68 000 and all residents are assumed to have been exposed (Luo et al., 2003). Additionally, the fibre was used in family-style production to manufacture asbestos products such as stoves, until banned in 1984. It is estimated that only about 50 people were involved in these activities (Lamb and Reid, 1968). The average number of mesothelioma cases diagnosed at a local county hospital was 6.6 per year from 1984-95, an incidence rate of 97 per million per year; and 22 per million per year from 1996 to 1999. The average annual mortality rates for mesothelioma determined from two cohort studies in the region was 85 per million per year during 1977-83 and 178 per million per year during 1987-95. The latter rate is lower but in the same order as the rate of 277 per million person-years (95% CI 170-384) found for mesothelioma in the mortality study of the birth cohort in the South African crocidolite mining district of Prieska (Kielkowski et al., 2000). Age-standardised mesothelioma incidence has been reported for past residents of Wittenoom without occupational exposure to asbestos (Hansen et al., 1998). At 260 per million person-years it is very similar to the Prieska rate. In central Anatolia, which had no occupational asbestos exposure, the standardised average annual mesothelioma rates were 114.8 per 100 000 (1148 per million) for men and 159.8 per 100 000 (1598 per million) for women (Metintas et al., 2002). These standardised Anatolia rates are considerably higher than those of Witternoom, and the highest environmental rates reported.

In contrast, studies of non-occupational mesothelioma in chrysotile mining regions are scanty and cases are rare in the few studies that have been published. For example, only seven deaths from pleural mesothelioma were identified in women living in the chrysotile mining areas of Thetford Mines and Asbestos, Quebec, Canada, during 1970 to 1989 (Camus et al., 1998). The combined population of the two towns was about 45 000 in 1981. At least three of the seven cases may have had occupational exposure to amphiboles (Churg, 1998). Balangero chrysotile mine in Italy was the largest in Europe and mined asbestos from 1917 to 1990 (Silvestri et al., 2001). The mine was surrounded by four municipalities which had a combined population of about 11 550 in 1991. Eight mesothelioma deaths were recorded in these residents during 1970-1988. Exposure histories were not reported. A further three cases were identified between 1990-1995 from one of the municipalities (unspecified) producing incidence rates of 1.86 per million person-years for men and 6.82 per million person-years for women. However, two of the cases probably had had occupational asbestos exposure (Silvestri et al., 2001). Asbest City in the Sverdlovsk region of the Russian Federation, contains the largest chrysotile mining and milling complex in the world (Scherbakov et al., 2001). Mining started in 1886. The city has had asbestos mills since the early 20th century and also had facilities for the manufacture of asbestos-containing goods. In 1999, Tomilova (see Scherbakov et al, 2001) reviewed 41 cases of mesothelioma that occurred in the Sverdlovsk region from 1981 to 1996. In 27% no history of occupational asbestos exposure was identified and in a further 34% no exposure data were available (Scherbakov et al., 2001). Five of the cases were from Asbest, producing a standardised incidence rate of 2.8 per million persons per year.

South Africa, like other countries that have mined and milled asbestos, has documented cases of mesothelioma attributable to environmental exposure. In South Africa the vast majority of these environmental cases can be attributed to exposure to Cape crocidolite. Large areas of the country particularly in the Northern Cape Province have been and remain heavily contaminated. Other areas of the country are also heavily contaminated with asbestos; for example, a report on the town of Penge suggests that the area has been found unfit for human habitation due to the ongoing dangers of asbestos pollution (Meintjes and Hermanus, 2008).

3. Conclusion

South Africa was a significant producer of crocidolite, amosite and chrysotile asbestos. From 1910 to 2002, a total of 10,099,568 tonnes of asbestos were mined. Local sales generated ZAR 1.746 billion and export sales ZAR 28.981 billion. In particular it supplied the world with crocidolite and amosite. The association between mesothelioma and asbestos was first described in South Africa, in individuals exposed occupationally and environmentally to Cape crocidolite. Cape crocidolite remains the most potent fibre type for the development of mesothelioma in South Africa for both occupationally and environmentally exposed people. The South African experience and the local research findings show that the association between Northern Cape crocidolite exposure and the development of mesothelioma is unequivocal.

While there have been cases of mesothelioma attributable to exposure to amosite in South Africa, the situation is clouded because of the possibility of mixed exposures to amosite and Transvaal crocidolite, both of which were mined in the Pietersburg asbestos field. There are very few studies of Transvaal crocidolite. The South African experience of a paucity of mesotheliomas attributable to pure amosite exposure appears to differ from that of countries which imported the fibre and used it industrially (Roggli et al., 1993; Gibbs and Berry, 2008). There is no satisfactory explanation for this difference. It is possible that the milled fibre behaves differently from the freshly mined fibre. Factors which add further uncertainty are under-ascertainment of cases due to the remoteness of the areas where mining took place, the poor quality of medical services in the labour-sending areas and widespread failure to report occupational disease.

In South Africa there are very few cases of mesothelioma that can be attributed to chrysotile. This is despite the fact that the commercial mining of chrysotile continued after the mining of crocidolite and amosite ceased. A possible explanation for this is that the amount of contamination of South African chrysotile with tremolite asbestos is very low (Rees et al., 2001). The mesotheliomagenic potential of South African chrysotile is certainly much less than that of Cape crocidolite and amosite.

Despite knowing about the adverse health effects of asbestos since 1928 (Simson, 1928) and its association with mesothelioma since 1960 (Wagner et al., 1960), asbestos mines continued to operate in South Africa until 2002. The closure of mines was more about the global market for asbestos than concerns for the health of the mine workers. Because of South Africa's past economic and political situation the mining companies had a great deal of influence (McCulloch, 2002). Pressure from the industry sought to limit research into the adverse health effects of asbestos and delayed the publication of reports and scientific studies, such as the PRU report and the Botha paper (PRU, 1964; Botha et al., 1986).

Data on exposure levels at South African mines and mills are sparse. Poor record keeping, variable criteria for measurement and changes in the instruments used for measuring dust and fibre levels contributed to this situation (Sluis-Cremer et al., 1992). Where data is available the exposure levels for workers were shown to be extremely high (Rendall and Davies, 2007). As a consequence, levels of benign pleural and parenchymal asbestos-related disease are high (Davies et al., 2001; Davies et al., 2004).

When the mines closed they left a legacy of disease and a contaminated environment. Litigation, class actions and eventually an out of court settlement resulted in the founding of the ART and KRT funds (KRT, 2011). These funds offered restitution in the form of compensation money to individuals and their families who suffered because of asbestos-related diseases. In terms of this settlement, compensation became available for the first time for environmentally exposed individuals. A small amount of money was also made available for rehabilitation of the environment. The money for the funds came from a number of companies that mined asbestos. Access to these funds and compensation was limited to ex-employees of these companies and individuals who lived in the vicinity of these mines. Not all mines were part of this settlement. A significant number of mines, mills, tailings dumps and surface workings are persistent sources of environmental contamination. Former workers at these operations are not covered by the trusts and cannot claim from them.

While the ART and KRT have done an excellent job in tracing, examining and compensating claimants, huge social and environmental problems persist. The contamination is not confined to the areas in the vicinity of mines. The transportation of asbestos contaminated other areas including railways, roads, marshalling yards, warehouses and docks (Braun and Kisting, 2006). Asbestos containing building materials pose an ongoing hazard for construction and demolition workers (Phillips et al., 2006; Phillips et al., 2007; Phillips et al., 2009). The disposal of asbestos containing material and the maintenance of asbestos dump sites is an ongoing problem. There is a shortage of housing and building materials in South Africa and the recycling of asbestos cement building materials, although banned in legislation, continues.

Despite being the world's largest producer of crocidolite and amosite, South African mesothelioma mortality rates for the period 1995 to 2007 are much lower than expected. In 1984, South Africa had one of the highest mesothelioma rates in the world. Unlike Australia where the rate of mesothelioma is still rising, the rate in South Africa appears to have peaked. The reasons for this are not entirely clear. It may be due to under reporting or competing causes of death related to the AIDS epidemic in the country (Kielkowski et al., 2011). In the 1950s, cases of mesothelioma were being mistaken for atypical pleural tuberculosis. Currently, tuberculosis is the most common AIDS defining illness in South Africa and co-infection is present in up to 80% of cases of tuberculosis. Given this background of a high mortality rate due to HIV/AIDS and tuberculosis, it is possible that cases of mesothelioma are being missed.

Although asbestos mining has ceased and the manufacture, import and export of asbestos containing products is banned, there is still a legacy of existing durable asbestos containing products in the environment (Braun and Kisting, 2006). Furthermore the asbestos deposits remain in the ground. Mining of minerals continues to be important to the economy of the country and asbestos deposits occur in association with other mineral deposits. In order to exploit the mineral wealth of South Africa, there is evidence of accidental or incidental mining of asbestos (Figure 9). In diamond mines the kimberlite ore body is drilled dry. Asbestos is known to occur in association with kimberlite pipes and the incidental mining of asbestos can occur. A risk of exposure to asbestos has recently been shown in a study of South African diamond miners. Tremolite-actinolite asbestos fibres have been identified in the lungs of miners and in the tailings from diamond mines. In this retrospective autopsy-based study of diamond miners, asbestosis, pleural plaques, a lung cancer and a case of mesothelioma were identified (Nelson et al., 2011).

Looking back on the South African experience with asbestos, it is clear that there were lessons that should have been learned sooner. The collection of data about exposure in the workplace and in the environment is vital. The analysis of these data leads to conclusions that should be incorporated into policy and implemented (Murray et al., 2011). On the whole, this has not been the case in the South African mining industry.

The question needs to be asked: on balance, was it worth mining asbestos? The commercial advantage never amounted to more than 3% of the total value of mineral- based revenues

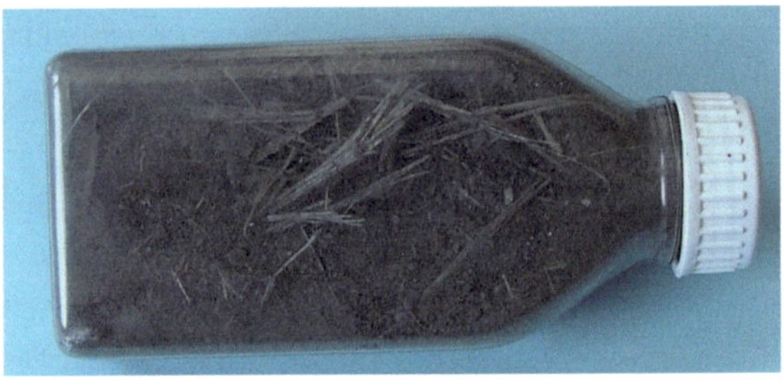

Figure 9. Tremolite asbestos fibres from the tailings dump of South African platinum mine. (Courtesy of Professor JI Phillips).

generated by the mining industry. It is impossible to put a value on the pain and suffering due to asbestos-related disease. Money has been spent on health care and compensation, and more will need to be spent. Similarly, money has been spent on rehabilitation of the environment but much more needs to be spent on cleaning up vast tracks of land, including roads and railways as well as the remediation of old mining areas and the maintenance of asbestos waste dumps.

Author details

James I. Phillips
National Institute for Occupational Health, National Health Laboratory Service, South Africa
Deparatment of Biomedical Technology, Faculty of Health Sciences, University of Johannesburg, South Africa

David Rees, Jill Murray and John C.A. Davies
National Institute for Occupational Health, National Health Laboratory Service, South Africa
School of Public Health, Faculty of Health Sciences, University of the Witwatersrand, South Africa

Acknowledgement

The authors would like to acknowledge the many members of the staff of the NIOH, both past and present, who contributed to this work. The contribution of Prof JI Phillips is based on research supported by the National Research Foundation.

4. References

Abratt RP, Vorobiof DA, White N. 2004. Asbestos and mesothelioma in South Africa. Lung Cancer 45 Suppl 1:S3-6.

Becklake MR, Case BW. 1994. Fiber burden and asbestos-related lung disease: determinants of dose-response relationships. Am J Respir Crit Care Med 150:1488-1492.

Botha JL, Irwig LM, Strebel PM. 1986. Excess mortality from stomach cancer, lung cancer, and asbestosis and/or mesothelioma in crocidolite mining districts in South Africa. Am J Epidemiol 123:30-40.

Braun L, Kisting S. 2006. Asbestos-related disease in South Africa: the social production of an invisible epidemic. Am J Public Health 96:1386-1396.

Camus M, Siemiatycki J, Meek B. 1998. Nonoccupational exposure to chrysotile asbestos and the risk of lung cancer. N Engl J Med 338:1565-1571.

Churg A. 1988. Chrysotile, tremolite, and malignant mesothelioma in man. Chest 93:621-628.

Churg A. 1994. Deposition and clearance of chrysotile asbestos. Ann Occup Hyg 38:625-633, 424-625.

Churg A. 1998. Nonoccupational exposure to chrysotile asbestos and the risk of lung cancer. N Engl J Med 339:999; author reply 1001-1002.

Cochrane JC, Webster I. 1978. Mesothelioma in relation to asbestos fibre exposure. A review of 70 serial cases. S Afr Med J 54:279-281.

Coetzee CB, Brabers AJM, Malherbe SJ, van Biljon WJ. 1976. Asbestos: Mineral Resources of the Republic of South Africa. Department of Mines, Geological Survey. Government Printer, Pretoria. ISBN 0 621 03464 9.

Davies JC, Kielkowski D, Phillips JI, Govuzela M, Solomon A, Makofane MR, Sekgobela ML, Garton E. 2004. Asbestos in the sputum, crackles in the lungs, and radiologic changes in women exposed to asbestos. Int J Occup Environ Health 10:220-225.

Davies JC, Williams BG, Debeila MA, Davies DA. 2001. Asbestos related lung disease among women in the Northern Province of South Africa. S Afr J Sci 97:87-92.

Davies JCA, Landau SP, Goldsmith C, Langton ME. 1987. Mesothelioma risk among gold miners in South Africa. South African Journal of Science 83:184-185.

du Toit RS. 1992. Dust survey. Internal report. Rdt 4.13.16.

Edginton ME, Hodkinson J, Seftel HC. 1972. Disease patterns in a South African rural Bantu population, including a commentary on comparisons with the pattern in urbanized Johannesburg Bantu. S Afr Med J 46:968-976.

Egilman D, Fehnel C, Bohme SR. 2003. Exposing the "myth" of ABC, "anything but chrysotile": a critique of the Canadian asbestos mining industry and McGill University chrysotile studies. Am J Ind Med 44:540-557.

Felix MA. 1997. Environmental asbestos and respiratory disease in South Africa. Ph.D Thesis, Faculty of Medicine. University of the Witwatersrand, Johannesburg. p 281.

Felix MA, Leger J, Ehrlich RI. 1994. Three minerals, three epidemics - asbestos mining and disease in South Africa. Advances in Modern Environmental Toxicology 21.

Gibbs GW, Berry G. 2008. Mesothelioma and asbestos. Regul Toxicol Pharmacol 52:S223-231.

Hansen J, de Klerk NH, Musk AW, Hobbs MS. 1998. Environmental exposure to crocidolite and mesothelioma: exposure-response relationships. Am J Respir Crit Care Med 157:69-75.

Harington JS, McGlashan ND. 1998. South African asbestos: production, exports, and destinations, 1959-1993. Am J Ind Med 33:321-326.

Harington JS, McGlashan ND, Chelkowska EZ. 2010. South Africa's export trade in asbestos: demise of an industry. Am J Ind Med 53:524-534.

Hart HP. 1988. Asbestos in South Africa. J. S. Afr. Inst. Min. Metall. 88:185-198.

Hodgson JT, McElvenny DM, Darnton AJ, Price MJ, Peto J. 2005. The expected burden of mesothelioma mortality in Great Britain from 2002 to 2050. Br J Cancer 92:587-593.

Huncharek M. 1994. Asbestos and cancer: epidemiological and public health controversies. Cancer Invest 12:214-222.

Kielkowski D, Nelson G, Bello B, Kgalamono S, Phillips JI. 2011. Trends in mesothelioma mortality rates in South Africa: 1995-2007. Occup Environ Med 68:547-549.

Kielkowski D, Nelson G, Rees D. 2000. Risk of mesothelioma from exposure to crocidolite asbestos: a 1995 update of a South African mortality study. Occup Environ Med 57:563-567.

KRT 2011. Annual Report. Asbestos Relief Trust. URL http://www.asbestostrust.co.za/ (accessed 21/6/2012).

Lamb D, Reid L. 1968. Mitotic rates, goblet cell increase and histochemical changes in mucus in rat bronchial epithelium during exposure to sulphur dioxide. J Pathol Bacteriol 96:97-111.

Langer AM, Nolan RP. 1994. Chrysotile biopersistence in the lungs of persons in the general population and exposed workers. Environ Health Perspect 102 Suppl 5:235-239.

Langer AM, Selikoff IJ, Sastre A. 1971. Chrysotile asbestos in the lungs of persons in New York City. Arch Environ Health 22:348-361.

Luo S, Liu X, Mu S, Tsai SP, Wen CP. 2003. Asbestos related diseases from environmental exposure to crocidolite in Da-yao, China. I. Review of exposure and epidemiological data. Occup Environ Med 60:35-41; discussion 41-32.

Malherbe HH. 1974. The viruses of vervet monkeys and of baboons in South Africa. M.D. Thesis, Faculty of Medicine. University of the Witwatersrand, Johannesburg. p 65.

Manfredi JJ, Dong J, Liu WJ, Resnick-Silverman L, Qiao R, Chahinian P, Saric M, Gibbs AR, Phillips JI, Murray J, Axten CW, Nolan RP, Aaronson SA. 2005. Evidence against a role for SV40 in human mesothelioma. Cancer Res 65:2602-2609.

Martiny O. 1956. Primary mesothelioma of the pleura. Proc. Transvaal Mine Medical Officers' Assoc. 35:63-64.

McCulloch J. 2002. Asbestos Blues. Oxford and Indianapolis: James Currey and Indiana University Press.

McCulloch J. 2003. Asbestos mining in Southern Africa, 1893-2002. Int J Occup Environ Health 9:230-235.

McDonald JC. 2010. Epidemiology of malignant mesothelioma--an outline. Ann Occup Hyg 54:851-857.

Meintjes S, Hermanus M. 2008. "Unfit for human habitation: The Penge report". In: Phiroshaw C, editor. National Asbestos Conference Report, ISBN: 978-0-620-46691-2 ed. Johannesburg: KRT and ART. p 55-59.

Metintas S, Metintas M, Ucgun I, Oner U. 2002. Malignant mesothelioma due to environmental exposure to asbestos: follow-up of a Turkish cohort living in a rural area. Chest 122:2224-2229.

Mothemela M. 2011. Mesothelioma in South Africa three decades post peak of asbestos production: an analysis of claims database of asbestos ex-miners. In: African regional association of occupational health congress: Care for the occupational health needs of the worker. Birchwood Hotel, Boksburg, South Africa. URL http://www.asbestostrust.co.za/documents/Abstracts-2011.pdf (accessed 21/6/2012)

Murray J, Davies JCA, Rees D. 2011. Occupational lung disease in the South African mining industry: Research and policy implementation. Journal of Public Health Policy 32:S65-S79.

Murray J, Nelson G. 2008. Health effects of amosite mining and milling in South Africa. Regul Toxicol Pharmacol 52:S75-81.

Nelson G, Murray J, Phillips JI. 2011. The risk of asbestos exposure in South African diamond mine workers. Ann Occup Hyg 55:569-577.

Nishikawa K, Takahashi K, Karjalainen A, Wen CP, Furuya S, Hoshuyama T, Todoroki M, Kiyomoto Y, Wilson D, Higashi T, Ohtaki M, Pan G, Wagner G. 2008. Recent mortality from pleural mesothelioma, historical patterns of asbestos use, and adoption of bans: a global assessment. Environ Health Perspect 116:1675-1680.

Nolan RP, Ross M, Nord GL, Raskina M, Phillips JI, Murray, J, Gibbs GW. 2006. Asbestos Fibre-type and Mesothelioma Risk in the Republic of South africa. Clay Science 12:223 - 227.

Phillips JI, Murray J. 2009. South African data on malignant mesothelioma. Ind Health 47:198-199.

Phillips JI, Norman G, Renton K. 2009. Asbestos in soil around dwellings in Soweto. Occupational Health Southern Africa 15:24-27.

Phillips JI, Renton K, Badenhorst C. 2006. Potential health hazard from cleaning asbestos cement roofs: A case report. Occup Health Southern Africa 12:20-22.

Phillips JI, Renton K, Murray J, Garton E, Tylee BE, Rees D. 2007. Asbestos in and around Soweto dwellings with asbestos roofs. Occupational Health Southern Africa 13:3 - 7.

PRU. 1964. Field survey in the North Western Cape and at Penge in the Transvaal. In. Johannesburg: Pneumoconiosis Research Unit. p 64.

Public-Protector SA. 2008. Report on an investigation into allegations of an improper insistence on the provision of documentary proof of service relating to claims for benefits and an improper refusal to accept affidavits by the Compensation Commissioner for Occupational Diseases. In. p 29.

Rees D, du Toit RSJ, Rendall REG, van Sittert GCH, Rama DBK. 1992. Tremolite in South African chrysotile. S Afr J Sci 88:468-469.

Rees D, Goodman K, Fourie E, Chapman R, Blignaut C, Bachmann MO, Myers J. 1999a. Asbestos exposure and mesothelioma in South Africa. S Afr Med J 89:627-634.

Rees D, Myers JE, Goodman K, Fourie E, Blignaut C, Chapman R, Bachmann MO. 1999b. Case-control study of mesothelioma in South Africa. Am J Ind Med 35:213-222.

Rees D, Phillips JI, Garton E, Pooley FD. 2001. Asbestos lung fibre concentrations in South African chrysotile mine workers. Ann Occup Hyg 45:473-477.

Rees DJ. 1995. A case-control study of mesothelioma in South Africa. Ph.D. Thesis, Faculty of Medicine. University of Cape Town. p 192.

Reid G, Kielkowski D, Steyn SD, Botha K. 1990. Mortality of an asbestos-exposed birth cohort. A pilot study. S Afr Med J 78:584-586.

Rendall RE. 1980. Physical and chemical characteristics of UICC reference samples. IARC Sci Publ: 30:87-96

Rendall REG, Davies JCA. 2007. Dust and fibre levels at Penge amosite mine 1970 to 1971. Adler Mus Bull 33:26-30.

Rogers A, Nevill M. 1995. Occupational and environmental mesotheliomas due to crocidolite mining activities in Wittenoom, Western Australia. Scand J Work Environ Health 21:259-264.

Roggli VL, Pratt PC, Brody AR. 1993. Asbestos fiber type in malignant mesothelioma: an analytical scanning electron microscopic study of 94 cases. Am J Ind Med 23:605-614.

Scherbakov SV, Kashansky S, Domnin SG, Koslov V, Kochelayev VA, Nolan RP. 2001. The health effects of mining and milling chrysotile: The Russian experience.: Mineralogical Association of Canada.

Silvestri S, Magnani C, Calisti R, Bruno C. 2001. The experience of the Balangero chrysotile mine in Italy: Health effects among workers mining and milling asbestos and the health experience of persons living nearby.: Mineralogical Association of Canada.

Simson FW. 1928. Pulmonary asbestosis in South Africa. BMJ 1:885-887.

Slade GF. 1931. The incidence of respiratory disability in workers employed in asbestos mining, with special reference to the type of disability caused by the inhalation of asbestos dust. In. Johannesburg: University of the Witwatersrand. p 150.

Sleggs CA, Marchand P, Wagner C. 1961. Diffuse pleural mesothelioma in South Africa. South African Medical journal 35:28 - 34.

Sluis-Cremer GK. 1965. Asbestosis in South Africa--certain geographical and environmental considerations. Ann N Y Acad Sci 132:215-234.

Sluis-Cremer GK. 1970. Asbestosis in South African asbestos miners. Environ Res 3:310-319.

Sluis-Cremer GK, Liddell FD, Logan WP, Bezuidenhout BN. 1992. The mortality of amphibole miners in South Africa, 1946-80. Br J Ind Med 49:566-575.

Smith AH, Wright CC. 1996. Chrysotile asbestos is the main cause of pleural mesothelioma. Am J Ind Med 30:252-266.

Solomons K. 1984. Malignant mesothelioma--clinical and epidemiological features. A report of 80 cases. S Afr Med J 66:407-412.

Stayner LT, Dankovic DA, Lemen RA. 1996. Occupational exposure to chrysotile asbestos and cancer risk: a review of the amphibole hypothesis. Am J Public Health 86:179-186.

Talent JM, Harrison WO, Webster I. 1978. The prevalence of asbestosis, pleural changes and malignant neoplasia in black ex-miners and female cobbers. In: Annual Report. Johannesburg: National Research Institute for Occupational Diseases. p 36 -37.

Timbrell V, Rendall RE. 1971. Preparation of the UICC Standard Reference Samples of asbestos. Powder Technology 5:279-287.

Virta RL. 2006. Worldwide asbestos supply and consumption trends from 1900 through 2003: US Geological Survey circular 1298, 80p. In.

Wagner JC. 1962. The pathology of asbestosis in South Africa. M.D. Thesis, School of Pathology, University of the Witwatersrand, Johannesburg. p 150.

Wagner JC. 1986. Mesothelioma and mineral fibers. Cancer 57:1905-1911.

Wagner JC. 1991. The discovery of the association between blue asbestos and mesotheliomas and the aftermath. Br J Ind Med 48:399-403.

Wagner JC, Sleggs CA, Marchand P. 1960. Diffuse pleural mesothelioma and asbestos exposure in the North Western Cape Province. Br J Ind Med 17:260-271.

Webster I. 1973. Asbestos and malignancy. S Afr Med J 47:165-171.

Webster I, Goldstein B, Coetzee FS, van Sittert GC. 1993. Malignant mesothelioma induced in baboons by inhalation of amosite asbestos. Am J Ind Med 24:659-666.

White N, Nelson G, Murray J. 2008. South African experience with asbestos related environmental mesothelioma: is asbestos fiber type important? Regul Toxicol Pharmacol 52:S92-96.

Zwi AB, Reid G, Landau SP, Kielkowski D, Sitas P, Becklake MR. 1989. Mesothelioma in South Africa, 1976-84: incidence and case characteristics. Int J Epidemiol 18:320-329.

Chapter 2

Effect of Asbestos on Anti-Tumor Immunity and Immunological Alteration in Patients with Malignant Mesothelioma

Yasumitsu Nishimura, Megumi Maeda, Naoko Kumagai-Takei, Hidenori Matsuzaki, Suni Lee, Kazuya Fukuoka, Takashi Nakano, Takumi Kishimoto and Takemi Otsuki

Additional information is available at the end of the chapter

http://dx.doi.org/10.5772/33138

1. Introduction

It is well known that malignant mesothelioma is caused by exposure to asbestos, which comprises a group of naturally occurring fibrous minerals. However, the mechanism by which asbestos causes malignant mesothelioma remains unclear. Many researchers have examined the effect of exposure to asbestos on the body. To date, it has been confirmed that asbestos can cause various forms of damage to cells, including cellular toxicity and mutagenicity, as well as produce reactive oxygen species (ROS) (Mossman & Churg, 1998; Mossman et al., 1996; Sporn & Roggli, 2004). The levels of oxidized pyrimidine and alkylated bases correlate with the period of occupational exposure to asbestos (Dusinska et al., 2004), and the increase in mutation frequency of lung DNA is caused by instillation of asbestos through the trachea (Topinka et al., 2004). All of these factors are thought to generate the tumorigenic effect of asbestos on mesothelial cells. However, the development of malignant mesothelioma caused by exposure to asbestos shows the noteworthy characteristics of this condition, which differ from those induced by other toxic materials. Malignant mesothelioma develops under a relatively low or medium dose of exposure to asbestos. A high dose of exposure to asbestos causes the development of pneumoconiosis, i.e., asbestosis rather than mesothelioma. Thus, the development of mesothelioma caused by exposure to asbestos cannot be explained only by a general rule regarding a dose-response relationship of toxic materials. In addition, it takes a long period of about forty years to develop malignant mesothelioma after exposure to asbestos. These findings suggest the existence of other factors related to the development of malignant mesothelioma that are modified by exposure to asbestos in the body, and which differ from the well-known tumorigenic effect of asbestos on mesothelial cells. One possible factor seems to be the effect of exposure to asbestos on anti-tumor immunity. In the body, the development of tumors is protected by anti-tumor immunity, composed of various kinds of cells including dendritic cells (DC), natural killer (NK) cells, helper T (Th) cells, cytotoxic T lymphocytes (CTLs), and so on. Exposure to asbestos might cause a suppressive effect on anti-tumor immunity in addition to the tumorigenic effect on mesothelial cells, and the combination of immune-suppressive and tumorigenic effects of asbestos might contribute to the development of malignant tumor (Fig. 1).

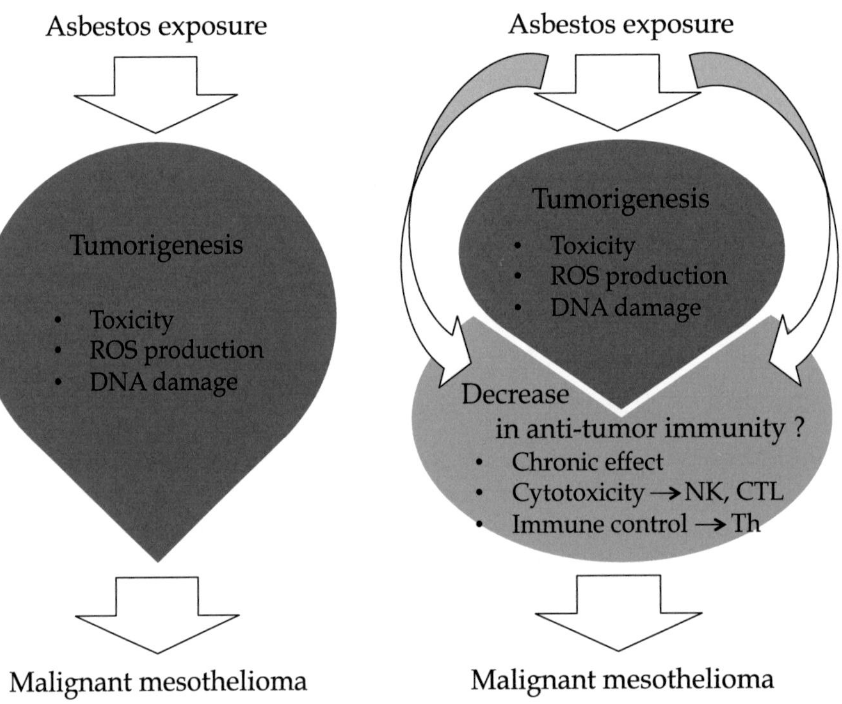

Figure 1. Hypothesis concerning the development of malignant mesothelioma caused by the immunological and tumorigenic effects of asbestos exposure. Many researchers have attempted to examine the tumorigenic effect of asbestos, thought to cause malignant mesothelioma (left). We propose the hypothesis that immune-suppressive effects, including the effect on NK- and T-cell functions, and the tumorigenic effects of asbestos exposure might contribute to the development of malignant mesothelioma (right).

The lung is not the only place where immune competent cells are able to meet asbestos fibers. Inhaled asbestos fibers reach the lung via the trachea, but they do not remain at that site. Those fibers translocate into the lung-draining lymph nodes over a long period. Dodson et al. examined the amount of asbestos in the lungs, lymph nodes, and plaque in a cohort of former shipyard workers, and reported that an analysis of asbestos in the lymph nodes confirmed accumulation in these sites (Dodson et al., 1991). In addition, asbestos fibers in the lymph nodes can translocate into the blood and may be observed in any tissue of the body, even in the brain where the accumulation of asbestos is low because of the blood-brain barrier (Miserocchi et al., 2008). Thus, immune competent cells have many opportunities to encounter asbestos fibers in the body, and the primary place where these cells meet asbestos seems to be the lung-draining lymph nodes (Fig. 2).

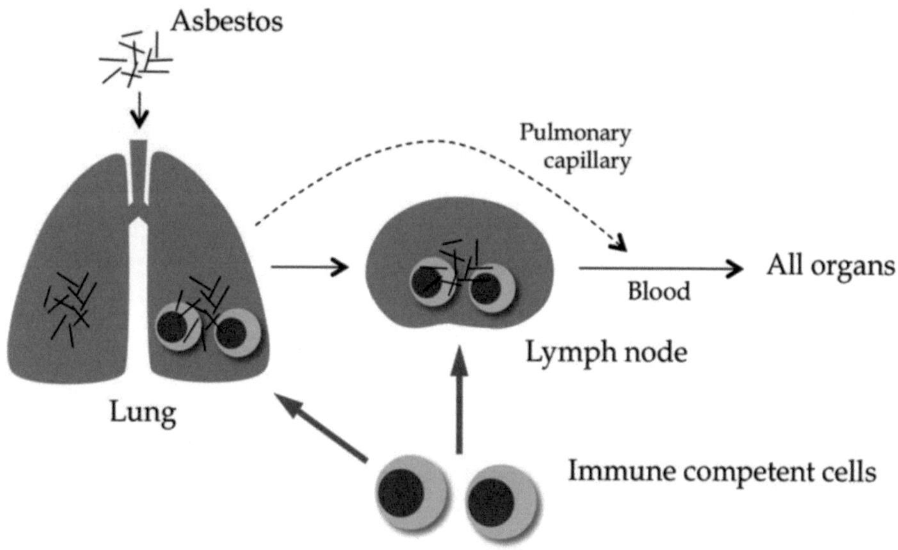

Figure 2. Places where immune competent cells encounter asbestos. Inhaled asbestos fibers reach the lung and translocate into the lung-draining lymph nodes. Therefore, the primary places where immune cells encounter asbestos seem to be the lung-draining lymph nodes.

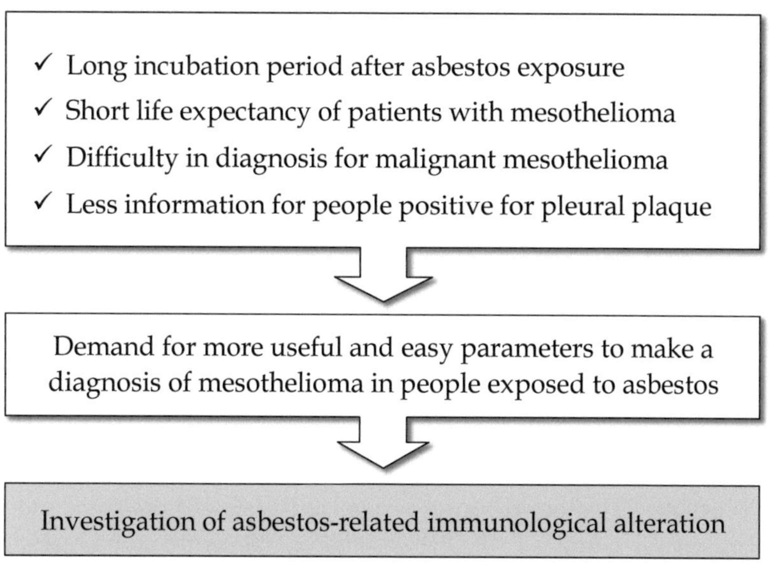

Figure 3. Present problems in malignant mesothelioma and the demand for a new parameter useful in making a diagnosis of malignant mesothelioma. Due to the problems shown in the top box, more useful and easy parameters to detect malignant mesothelioma in people exposed to asbestos are needed, to which our investigation of asbestos-related immunological alteration might contribute.

The present diagnosis for malignant mesothelioma is based on X-ray and CT image analyses, as well as pathohistological analysis. However, diagnosis using these procedures is sometimes accompanied with a risk of radiation exposure or invasiveness, and results are not regarded equally among doctors because they have learned these analyses separately and it is not easy to master all of these methods. In addition, although it takes a long period to develop malignant mesothelioma after exposure to asbestos, the mean life expectancy of patients with malignant mesothelioma is short, and people exposed to asbestos need a safer analysis that can be used frequently in a year in order to detect malignant mesothelioma as early as possible. Recently, the use of products derived from mesothelioma cells for diagnosis has been proposed, including megakaryocyte potentiating factor (MPF) and mesothelin (Creaney et al., 2007; Onda et al., 2006). However, those products might not be observed in the blood that early because they will appear exactly after the development of mesothelioma, and it may take some time for those products to transfer from the pleural cavity into the blood stream. Many people exposed to asbestos worry about the development of malignant mesothelioma; however, there is little predictive information regarding the onset of mesothelioma. Therefore, there is a need to find a new parameter or method useful for the early diagnosis of malignant mesothelioma (Fig. 3). If some characteristic alteration of immune function is caused by exposure to asbestos that is also found in patients with malignant mesothelioma, which can be measured by checking lymphocytes or other cells in peripheral blood, the analysis for that alteration might contribute to the early detection of malignant mesothelioma.

On the basis of these ideas, we started to investigate the immunological effect of exposure to asbestos and immunological alteration in patients with malignant mesothelioma. In this chapter, we show the results obtained from these studies concerning the effect of asbestos on anti-tumor immunity, focusing on NK and Th cells, and discuss the immune-suppressive effect of asbestos and the possible application of our results for the early diagnosis of malignant mesothelioma.

2. NK cells

The role in cytotoxicity against target cells in anti-tumor immunity is played by two populations of cells, natural killer (NK) cells and cytotoxic T lymphocytes (CTLs). NK cells have a cytotoxicity for targets which they are ready to kill without prior stimulation, whereas this readiness is absent from the killing activity of CTLs and is induced by antigen stimulation. Therefore, although the cytotoxicity of NK cells has no antigen specificity, it is thought to contribute widely to the early deletion of unhealthy cells such as virus-infected cells or transformed cells. On the other hand, it takes time to induce the differentiation of naïve $CD8^{+}$ T cells to CTLs, but they can recognize target cells precisely and injure them effectively. Imai et al. examined whether differences between individuals in regard to natural immunological host defense, i.e., NK cytotoxicity, can predict the future development of cancer. They reported that medium and high cytotoxic activity of peripheral blood lymphocytes is associated with reduced cancer risk, whereas low activity is associated with increased cancer risk, and these findings suggest a role for natural immunological host defense mechanisms against cancer (Imai et al., 2000). Therefore, we examined the effect of exposure to asbestos on cytotoxicity of NK cells and alteration in cytotoxicity of NK cells in patients with malignant mesothelioma.

2.1. Mechanism of cytotoxicity in NK cells

The mechanism of cytotoxicity in NK cells and CTLs can be separated into two parts. The role of one part is to recognize target cells, which is followed by transduction of the stimulation signal into the cytosol, while the other part acts to kill target cells. In the killing mechanism, both NK cells and CTLs use the common molecules perforin and granzymes. Perforin- and granzyme-induced apoptosis is the main pathway used by cytotoxic lymphocytes to eliminate virus-infected or transformed cells (Trapani & Smyth, 2002). Perforin and granzymes are produced and accumulate in the cytotoxic granules of NK cells. Once NK cells are optimally stimulated, perforin and granzymes are released into the gap of the immune synapse by degranulation and act on target cells to induce apoptosis. Perforin is the protein that can disrupt the cellular membrane and create a pore in the membrane of the target cell. Granzyme is a family of structurally related serine proteases, which enters target cells through the pore made by perforin, and induces apoptosis of the target cells. The second pathway to kill targets is Fas-mediated apoptosis, induced by ligation of the Fas ligand (FasL) expressed on NK cells or CTLs with Fas on target cells. In addition to these two pathways, tumor-necrosis factor-related apoptosis-inducing ligand (TRAIL) is also known to control the growth and metastasis of tumors (Smyth et al., 2001; Takeda et al., 2001). These killing mechanisms are followed by recognition of target cells by NK cells. In contrast to T cell, which utilizes the T cell receptor (TCR) to recognize targets, NK cells utilize various kinds of receptors for target recognition. These receptors could be of either type: inhibitory or activating. In the next section, we explain the significance of the expression levels of NK cell receptors for cytolytic activity.

2.2. NK cell receptors

NK cells do not have clonal diversity like T cells, which include many repertoires, rearrangements, and somatic mutations of TCRs. However, NK cells can recognize various target cells using various kinds of receptors expressed on the cell surface of NK cells (Moretta, L. & Moretta, A., 2004; Yokoyama & Plougastel, 2003). Some NK cell receptors, the ligands of which are human leukocyte antigen (HLA) molecules, genetically differing among individuals and recognized by T cells with T cell receptor (TCR) to find abnormal cells, have the role of transducing an inhibitory signal. Those inhibitory receptors include a KIR family of receptors and heterodimer of NKG2A and CD94. The inhibitory signals derived from those receptors contribute to prohibition of cytotoxicity against normal self cells. In contrast, several other receptors transduce an activation signal after ligation with their respective ligands to induce cytotoxicity against abnormal target cells (Fig. 4). NKG2D is the best characterized activating receptor expressed on NK cells. NKG2D is a receptor belonging to the same group as NKG2A, NKG2 family, characterized by a lectin-like domain, but can transduce an activation signal unlike NKG2A. The signaling lymphocytic activation molecule (SLAM) family is another group of activating receptors expressed on NK cells. A representative receptor of the SLAM family is 2B4, which induces cytotoxicity by stimulation with the natural ligand, CD48, or the antibody to 2B4 (Endt et al., 2007; Garni-Wagner et al., 1993; Valiante & Trinchieri, 1993). Moreover, natural cytotoxicity receptors (NCRs) make a family of receptors that includes NKp46, NKp44 and NKp30, which play a major role in the NK-mediated killing of most tumor cells (Moretta, A. et al., 2001; Sivori et al., 1999). These activating receptors transduce the stimulation signal leading to the phosphorylation of c-Jun N-terminal kinases (JNKs) and extracellular signal-regulated kinase (ERK), which cause polarization of the microtubule organizing center (MTOC) and cytotoxic granules followed by release of perforin and granzymes, producing degranulation (Chen et al., 2006; Chen et al., 2007). Thus, the various kinds of receptors expressed on NK cells control induction of cytotoxicity for target cells, and alteration in expression of these receptors is thought to affect the strength of the stimulation signal to induce cytotoxicity of NK cells. In addition, if NK cells exposed to asbestos show some characteristic alteration in expression of NK cell receptors, this alteration might be used as a possible marker of asbestos exposure-related immune alteration. Therefore, we planned to study the effect of asbestos exposure on NK cells, focusing on the expression level of NK cell receptors, as well as investigate the cytotoxicity of NK cells.

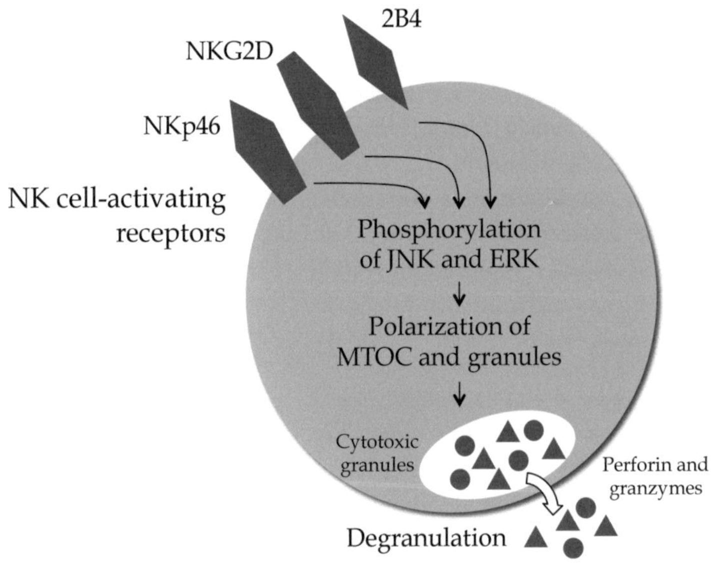

Figure 4. NK cell-activating receptors and the machinery of degranulation caused by stimulation with these receptors. The ligation of NK cell-activating receptors with their respective ligands induce phosphorylation of JNK and ERK, leading to polarization of the microtubule organizing center (MTOC) and granules, where perforin and granzymes are released and induce apoptosis of target cells.

2.3. Cytotoxicity of human NK cell line cultured with asbestos for a long period

We initially started by making the sub-line of an NK cell line by culturing cells exposed to asbestos for a long period. The human NK cell line of YT-A1 was kindly provided by Dr.

Yodoi and was used for this experiment. Before starting the culture, the effect of exposure to chrysotile B (CB) on the survival and growth of YT-A1 cells was examined in order to avoid a high dose of exposure to CB which induces intense apoptosis and inhibition of cell growth. The apoptosis of YT-A1 was not induced upon exposure to CB at concentrations from 5 to 100 μg/ml. However, cell growth was inhibited upon exposure to CB at a concentration greater than 50 μg/ml, whereas it was not inhibited below 20 μg/ml. Therefore, the dose of CB used was defined as 5 μg/ml, representing the concentration at which YT-A1 cells were cultured with CB, named YT-CB5, and the rest of cells was cultured in the original condition of media without CB, named YT-Org. The cultures were exposed for over five months and then periodically examined for the effect of asbestos exposure on the cytotoxicity of NK cells. The cells were assayed for cytotoxicity against K562 cells and expression levels of various kinds of NK cell receptors and other molecules using flow cytometry. There were no differences in cytotoxicity or expression levels of cell-surface molecules between YT-Org and YT-CB5 for one month after exposure to CB. However, after around 5 months of such exposure, YT-CB5 showed a clear decrease in cytotoxicity compared with YT-Org. In addition, decreases in expression levels of NKG2D and 2B4, but not of NKp46, were also found in YT-CB5 (Nishimura et al., 2009b). The expression level of CD56 and CD16, NK-cell marker and low-affinity Fc receptor, respectively, altered slightly. NKG2A, which makes a suppressive receptor with CD94, did not increase. In addition, YT-CB5 showed almost a zero level of granzyme A and exhibited a significant decrease in perforin, but the degree of decrease of perforin was not large and YT-CB5 did not show a significant decrease in granzyme B. Although 2B4 is not related to cytotoxicity against K562 cells in contrast to NKG2D and NKp46, YT-CB5 also showed the decrease in cytotoxicity against P815 cells treated with antibodies to 2B4, a cytotoxicity mediated by 2B4. These results supported the supposition that the decrease in NKG2D and 2B4 might cause impairment in induction of cytotoxicity by reducing signal transduction downstream of those receptors. Therefore, the degranulation stimulated by antibodies to NKG2D and 2B4 was examined in YT-CB5 by flow cytometry, which can estimate degranulation by measuring an increase in cell-surface CD107a accompanied with secretion of cytotoxic granules. YT-CB5 showed decreases in degranulation stimulated via NKG2D and 2B4, as observed under stimulation with bead-bound and plate-bound antibodies, respectively. In addition, YT-CB5 also showed a decrease in phosphorylation of ERK1/2 stimulated with K562 cells as well as antibodies to NKG2D, but not with antibodies to 2B4 (Nishimura et al., 2009a). Moreover, we examined cytotoxicity against K562 cells, expression levels of NKG2D, 2B4 and NKp46, and the phosphorylation level of ERK1/2 stimulated with their respective antibodies in peripheral blood (PB-) NK cells purified from the blood of healthy volunteers, and compared results among the volunteers. PB-NK cells with a high expression of NKG2D, derived from one individual, showed high cytotoxicity and high phosphorylation of ERK1/2, whereas both cytotoxicity and ERK phosphorylation were low in PB-NK cells with low NKG2D, derived from another individual. In a similar way, the relationship among the cell-surface level of NKp46, phosphorylation level of ERK1/2, and cytotoxicity was also investigated and confirmed in PB-NK cells of healthy volunteers. Thus, we demonstrated that exposure to asbestos caused an impairment in cytotoxicity of NK cells with decreases in NK cell-activating receptors. The decrease in NKG2D caused the low level of signal transduction, followed by a decrease in degranulation, in the asbestos-exposed subline of cells.

2.4. Low cytotoxicity and low NKp46 level in NK cells of mesothelioma patients

The result of the experiment using the human NK cell line described above suggested that inhaled asbestos might cause impairment in cytotoxicity with altered expression of NK cell-activating receptors, and that PB-NK cells in patients with malignant mesothelioma might show a similar impairment in cytotoxicity to YT-CB cells. Therefore, peripheral blood mononuclear cells (PBMCs) prepared from the blood of patients with mesothelioma were examined for cytotoxicity against K562 cells and expression levels of NKG2D, 2B4, and NKp46 in NK cells. The cytotoxicity of PBMCs against K562 in the tree different ratios of effector and targets was measured for each individual, and expressed as the percentage of specific lysis. To evaluate cytotoxicity per given number of NK cells, The number of NK cells in the cytotoxic reaction was calculated from the percentage of $CD3^{-}CD56^{+}$ NK cells in PBMCs and the number of PBMCs dispensed to each well of the culture plate for cytotoxic reaction. A linear regression line with the percentage of specific lysis and number of NK cells, in which the formula is *[percentage of specific lysis] = A [number of NK cells] + B*, was determined by using the three sets of percentage of specific lysis and number of NK cells for each individual. Finally, the percentages of specific lysis per 5000 NK cells from each individual were calculated from these regression lines and compared with those of healthy volunteers. Mesothelioma patients showed significantly lower cytotoxicity than healthy volunteers (Nishimura et al., 2009b). However, unlike YT-CB5, NK cells in patients with mesothelioma did not show a decrease in expression level of NKG2D or 2B4, whereas a decrease in NKp46 was observed in those NK cells. Thus, although NK cells in the peripheral blood of patients with malignant mesothelioma were not of the same character as YT-CB5, they also showed alteration in the expression of one of the NK-cell activating receptors, albeit a different one namely NKp46, with low expression of NKp46, and low cytotoxicity.

2.5. Low cytotoxicity of NK cells with low NKp46 in the culture of PBMCs with asbestos

As described above, NK cells in patients with malignant mesothelioma showed low cytotoxicity with low expression of NKp46, which was not found in YT-CB5. Therefore, to examine whether asbestos exposure causes such a decrease in NKp46 on NK cells, we performed a different experiment in which PBMCs from healthy volunteers were cultured in IL-2-supplemented media with chrysotile B at 5 μg/ml, and after 7 days cells were harvested and examined for expression levels of NKG2D, 2B4, and NKp46 in $CD3^{-}CD56^{+}$ NK cells by flow cytometry. IL-2 is a representative cytokine that induces proliferation and activation of NK cells and is commonly used to culture these cells. The results showed no decreases in cell-surface expression of NKG2D and 2B4 in NK cells derived from the culture with CB, whereas the expression of NKp46 decreased in those NK cells, resembling NK cells of patients with malignant mesothelioma (Nishimura et al., 2009b). To determine whether such restrictive alteration in expression of NK cell-activating receptors is caused by exposure to other mineral fibers, PBMCs were cultured with glass wool and then examined for the expression level of NKp46 on NK cells. Glass wool is a kind of man-made mineral fiber and is used as a representative substitute for asbestos. However, unlike asbestos, exposure to glass wool did not cause a decrease in expression of NKp46. These results indicate that exposure to asbestos causes the characteristic abnormality in human primary NK cells, resulting in a decrease in NKp46 but not in NKG2D. As described above, this characteristic is similar to that of PB-NK cells in patients with malignant mesothelioma, suggesting the possible relationship between asbestos exposure-related suppression of NK cell function and development of malignant mesothelioma.

3. $CD4^+$ T cells

What is the function of $CD4^+$ T cells in regard to an appropriate immune response? $CD4^+$ T cells, Th, contribute to various kinds of responses in innate and acquired immunity, including activation of NK cells, macrophages and dendritic cells (DC), as well as induction of antibody production and CTL development (Monney et al., 2002; Parker, 1993; Smith et al., 2004; Vivier et al., 2008). The production of various cytokines, including IL-2, IL-4, IL-5, IL-10, IL-17, IFN-γ, and TNF-α, by Th cells is one of the reasons for the multiple contributions of those cells to immune function (Fig. 5).

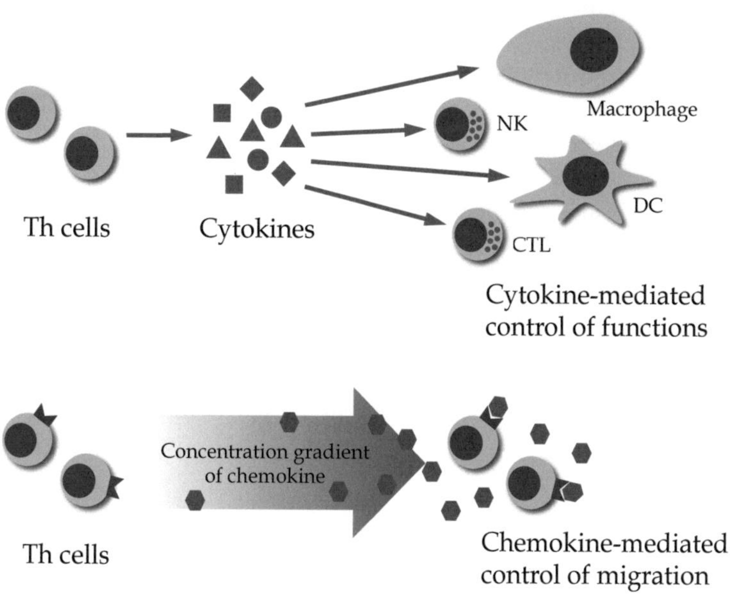

Figure 5. Cytokine-mediated control of immune functions and chemokine-mediated control of cell migration. The various kinds of cytokines produced by Th cells allow them to contribute widely to functions of immune competent cells (top). Concentration gradient of chemokines and expression of chemokine receptors play a key role in appropriate cell migration (bottom).

In addition, cytokines produced by Th cells can be transported by the blood stream, which allows them to exert an influence on distant cells as well as adjacent cells. Moreover, immune competent cells can migrate widely throughout the body, and Th cells are no exception to this rule. Chemokines, a group of cytokines, play a large role in such cell migration. For example, a chemokine produced in the periphery creates a concentration gradient, by which cells having the receptor for that chemokine can be attracted. Th cell migration is also controlled in a similar manner, in which the expression of receptors for chemokines influences the migration. As described below, our study discovered that the immunological effect of asbestos exposure involved a characteristic alteration in cytokine production and expression of chemokine receptor in Th cells chronically exposed to asbestos, and that Th cells in patients with malignant mesothelioma exhibited characteristics similar to those of asbestos-exposed cells. Before elaborating on these findings, in the next section we will detail the cytokines produced by Th cells and the Th cell migration controlled by chemokines and chemokine receptors.

3.1. Cytokines produced by Th cells and polarization to Th1, Th2, Treg and Th17 cells

Antigen stimulation, made by a complex of MHC class II and antigen peptide, allows naïve Th cells to proliferate and produce cytokines. Th cells produce various kinds of cytokines, which can be classified according to the role they have in immune functions. TNF-α and IFN-γ stimulate activation of NK cells and exert a promoting effect on the development of CTL, by which they support cell-mediated immunity for elimination of virus-infected or transformed/tumor cells. In contrast, IL-4 supports humoral immunity, in which it stimulates production of immunoglobulin, in particular IgE, by plasma cells differentiated from B cells, and is related to allergy and asthma. In addition, IFN-γ and IL-4 produced by Th cells show a mutual suppression in each other's production. As a result of such suppression, Th cells dominantly producing IFN-γ show less production of IL-4 and vice versa. Therefore, such development of Th cells exhibits a dominant production of cytokinesis, called "polarization", and the cells showing dominant production of IFN-γ and IL-4 are Th1 and Th2 cells, respectively (Liew, 2002). Moreover, part of the Th cells differentiate to regulatory T (Treg) cells, which dominantly produce IL-10 and TGF-β, immune-suppressive cytokines, and play a role in regulation of the immune response (Asseman et al., 1999; Dieckmann et al., 2002; Green et al., 2003; Jonuleit et al., 2002), although a part of Treg occurs naturally without antigen stimulation (Sakaguchi, 2005). It has also been reported that Th cells producing IL-17, called Th17, contribute to autoimmune diseases (Peck & Mellins, 2009). Thus, several cytokines produced by Th cells and subpopulations of polarized Th cells show a characteristic role in immune functions. Therefore, immune status can be estimated by examining the production of these cytokines.

3.2. Chemokine receptors expressed on Th cells

Although immune competent cells are spread over the body, they must move to the place where they are needed according to their functions, and this also applies to each subpopulation of Th cells. Naïve T cells, both $CD4^+$ and $CD8^+$ cells, have to reach secondary lymphoid organs to check an antigen processed by antigen-presenting cells. In contrast, Th1 and Th2 cells, as effector cells, move to the periphery where they must encounter appropriate partners. Therefore, the expression of receptors for chemokines differs among the subpopulations of Th cells (Sallusto & Lanzavecchia, 2000). Naïve T cells express the chemokine receptor CCR7, by which they acquire responsiveness to its ligands SLC and ELC and can move to secondary lymphoid organs. In contrast, Th1 and Th2 cells lose the expression of CCR7 and acquire the expression of CXCR3 and CCR5 or CCR3 and CCR4, respectively, although these expressions are a little flexible. CXCR3 is expressed on some NK cells, and CXCL10, the ligand of CXCR3, accumulates NK cells in tumors (Qin et al., 1998; Wendel et al., 2008). In addition, mice deficient for CXCL10 show impairment in T cell proliferation, IFN-γ production, contact hyper-sensitivity, a representative Th1 response, and recruitment of $CD4^+$ and $CD8^+$ cells in the periphery (Dufour et al., 2002). On the other hand, CCR3 is expressed at high levels on eosinophils, basophils, and mast cells, the population of cells related to allergy and asthma (Gerber et al., 1997). Thus, the subpopulations of Th cells differ in the expression of chemokine receptors, which is related to their different roles in immune functions, and the assay for expression of chemokine receptors on Th cells allows us to obtain information regarding the balance of the Th1/Th2 response as well as cell migration.

3.3. Impaired Th1 function of the human T cell line continuously exposed to asbestos

As described above, many immune functions are under the control of Th cells. Therefore, we examined the effect of asbestos exposure on Th cells. At the beginning of this study, we prepared an in vitro T-cell model of long-term and low-level exposure to chrysotile asbestos using MT-2 cells, a human adult T-cell leukemia virus (HTLV)-1-immortalized human polyclonal cell line, resulting in six sublines exposed to asbestos. These sublines were established from the independent cultures of MT-2 cells with chrysotile asbestos. All of the sublines acquired resistance to asbestos-induced apoptosis after more than eight months of continuous exposure, and were named MT-2Rsts. Those six MT-2Rsts were used for DNA microarray analysis, compared with the original MT-2 cells, named MT-2Org. The analysis clarified statistically significant alterations in expression of 139 genes in MT-2Rsts, greater than twofold changes. To identify genes related to the suppression of anti-tumor immunity, the expression data were processed by the MetaCore Analytical Suite (http://www.genego.com; GeneGo, St. Joseph, MI) to search for deregulated networks and pathways. The results obtained from pathway and network analysis showed down-regulation of IFN-γ signalling and CXCR3 expression in MT-2Rsts. As mentioned above, both IFN-γ and CXCR3 are related to Th1 cells. Therefore, we focused on Th1 functions of MT-2Rsts. All MT-2Rsts showed reduction of cell-surface expression of CXCR3, the mRNA level of which also decreased in MT-2Rsts, as assayed by real-time PCR. In addition, MT-2Rsts showed a decrease in production of IFN-γ compared to MT-2Org, as assayed by ELISA. Moreover, the production of CXCL10 also decreased in MT-2Rsts (Maeda et al.,

2010). These results indicate that continuous exposure of a human T cell line to asbestos impaired Th1 function, leading to decreases in cell-surface expression of CXCR3 and production of IFN-γ and CXCL10.

3.4. Decreases in CXCR3 and IFN-γ in primary $CD4^+$ T cells exposed to asbestos

Following the results obtained from the experiment using the MT-2 cell line, we examined the effect of asbestos exposure on human primary $CD4^+$ T cells (Maeda et al., 2011). $CD4^+$ T cells freshly isolated from PBMCs were stimulated with antibodies to CD3 and CD28 and cultured in IL-2-supplemented media for 3 days, and the activated $CD4^+$ T cells were transferred into a new culture plate and cultured with IL-2 for a week. These polyclonally expanded $CD4^+$ T cells were used for culture with chrysotile B asbestos. After 40 days of culture, cell surface CXCR3 expression decreased in a dose-dependent manner. In contrast, the expression of CCR5 varied among all healthy volunteers, and there were no significant changes after culture with chrysotile. In addition, we examined intracellular expression and the mRNA level of IFN-γ in $CD4^+$ T cells exposed to chrysotile B by flow cytometry and real-time PCR. The $CD4^+$ T cells exposed to chrysotile B showed a decrease in IFN-γ mRNA level, for which there was no significant difference, whereas IFN-γ positive cells tended to be reduced in those asbestos-exposed cells. These results indicate that chronic exposure to asbestos caused the decrease in CXCR3 and IFN-γ in $CD4^+$ T cells, in accordance with results obtained from the experiment using the cell line.

3.5. Decrease in $CD4^+CXCR3^+$ T cells in patients with mesothelioma

Finally, we determined whether $CD4^+$ T cells in asbestos-exposed patients showed the same impairment as shown by MT-2Rst sublines and in vitro asbestos-exposed primary $CD4^+$ T cells (Maeda et al., 2011). Individuals positive for pleural plaque and patients with malignant mesothelioma were examined for CXCR3 expression and IFN-γ production in peripheral blood $CD4^+$ T cells. Both plaque-positive individuals and mesothelioma patients showed a significantly lower percentage of $CXCR3^+$ cells in $CD4^+$ T cells than healthy volunteers. In addition, the percentages of $CD4^+$ $CXCR3^+$ T cells in lymphocytes from the plaque and mesothelioma groups were also significantly lower than those of the healthy group, and the mesothelioma group showed the lowest percentage among the three groups. In contrast to CXCR3, the percentage of $CCR5^+$ cells in $CD4^+$ T cells and $CD4^+$ $CCR5^+$ T cells in lymphocytes was not low in the plaque and mesothelioma groups. To examine production of IFN-γ by $CD4^+$ T cells from plaque-positive individuals and mesothelioma patients, $CD4^+$ T cells were stimulated with antibodies to CD3 and CD28, and cells and culture supernatants were harvested and assayed for mRNA and secreted levels of IFN-γ. The $CD4^+$ T cells of mesothelioma patients showed a significantly lower mRNA level of IFN-γ than that of plaque-positive individuals or healthy volunteers, whereas the secreted level of IFN-γ did not differ among the three groups. In addition, the concentration of CXCL10 in plasma tended to be higher for the plaque and mesothelioma groups than the healthy group, although there were no significant differences. CXCL10 can be produced by a variety of cells including endothelial cells, fibroblasts and monocytes near a cancerous lesion, to attract anti-tumor T cells (Luster & Ravetch, 1987; Dufour et al., 2002; Homey et al., 2002). Moreover, the mesothelioma group showed a tendency for an inverse correlation between the percentage of $CD4^{+}CXCR3^{+}$ T cells and CXCL10 concentration, in comparison with the plaque and healthy groups. These results indicate that anti-tumor immune function in mesothelioma patients may be in the situation with less recruitment of Th1 cells using CXCR3, although the level of its ligand, CXCL10, is high.

4. Conclusion and discussion

We examined the effect of asbestos exposure on NK-cell and Th-cell functions using human NK- and T-cell lines continuously exposed to asbestos, primary cell cultures with asbestos, and analyses for peripheral blood NK and Th cells in plaque-positive individuals and patients with malignant mesothelioma. The results obtained from these studies indicate that asbestos exposure causes functional alterations in NK and Th cells, decreases in cytotoxicity and expression of NKG2D or NKp46, and decreases in production of IFN-γ and expression of CXCR3, respectively. It is known that NK cell-activating receptors transduce a signal to induce phosphorylation of ERK and JNK, causing degranulation of cytotoxic granules. The results of our study also showed the relationship between the expression level of NKG2D or NKp46, ERK phosphorylation, and cytotoxicity using the NK cell line and peripheral blood NK cells from healthy individuals. Therefore, the asbestos-induced decrease in expression of NKG2D or NKp46 is thought to cause impairment of NK cell-mediated anti-tumor immunity. In addition, IFN-γ is a key cytokine for the Th1 response and CXCR3 is one of the representative chemokine receptors expressed on Th1 cells. Therefore, the asbestos-induced decrease of IFN-γ and CXCR3 in Th cells indicates the decrease of the Th1 response, which contributes to impairment of the immune response to tumors. These findings concerning NK and Th cells indicate that asbestos fibers have the potential to cause impairment of anti-tumor immunity. This is the first demonstration that asbestos exerts an immune suppressive effect, as well as a tumorigenic effect. The immune-suppressive effect of asbestos might contribute to development of malignant mesothelioma in people exposed to asbestos. As described in the introduction, asbestos is known to accumulate in the lung-draining lymph nodes, as well as the lungs, where NK and Th cells might be exposed to asbestos. Furthermore, the results of our studies indicate that several kinds of functional impairment in NK and Th cells observed in experiments of in vitro or ex vivo exposure to asbestos can also be observed in the cells of patients with malignant mesothelioma, although the results include some inconsistencies. NK cells in patients with mesothelioma showed the same decrease in NKp46 as NK cells in the PBMC culture with chrysotile asbestos, and Th cells in plaque-positive individuals and mesothelioma patients showed the same decrease in CXCR3 as the Th cell line and primary Th cells continuously cultured with chrysotile. In addition, it is noteworthy that there is also the consistency of parameters showing no alteration in expression between data from patients and cultures of primary cells. Those parameters are NKG2D and 2B4 for NK cells and CCR5 for Th cells, the altered expressions of which were not found in primary cells either exposed to asbestos or derived from patients with mesothelioma. These findings suggest that those characteristic functional alterations of NK and Th cells shown in patients with malignant mesothelioma might be caused by inhaled and accumulated asbestos in the body. Furthermore, they also suggest the possibility that decreases in NKp46 on NK cells and CXCR3 on Th cells might contribute to early diagnosis of malignant mesothelioma as markers to monitor asbestos-related immune suppression. Today, the diagnosis of malignant mesothelioma is dependent on X-ray and CT image analyses, as well as pathohistological analysis, but these procedures involve several problems such as difficulty in obtaining a consistent diagnosis and a risk of radiation exposure or invasiveness. In contrast, the drawing of blood necessary for analysis of immunological markers is safe and easy, and can be performed frequently during a year. Therefore, imaging and pathohistological analyses of malignant mesothelioma combined with immunological analysis for expression of NKp46 and CXCR3 might provide more valuable information for people who are exposed to asbestos and worry about the development of malignant mesothelioma. Further studies regarding the immunological effect of asbestos exposure will contribute to the effective diagnosis and therapy of malignant mesothelioma.

Acknowledgment

We thank Dr. Y. Yodoi for generously providing YT-Al cells, and Ms. Tamayo Hatayama, Satomi Hatada, Yoshiko Yamashita, Minako Kato, Tomoko Sueishi, Keiko Kimura, Misao Kuroki, Naomi Miyahara, and Shoko Yamamoto for their technical help. This study was supported by Special Coordination Funds for Promoting Science and Technology (H18-1-3-3-1), JSPS KAKENHI Grants (19790431, 18390186, 19659153, 19790411, 20890270, 20390178 and 22700933), The Takeda Science Foundation (Tokutei Kenkyu Josei I, 2008), Kawasaki Medical School Project Grants (18-209T, 19-407M, 19-603T, 19-205Y, 19-506, and 20-210O), and The Kawasaki Foundation for Medical Science and Medical Welfare (KYOIKU KENKYU JOSEI-2).

Author details

Yasumitsu Nishimura, Megumi Maeda,
Naoko Kumagai-Takei, Hidenori Matsuzaki, Suni Lee and Takemi Otsuki
Department of Hygiene, Kawasaki Medical School, Japan

Megumi Maeda
Division of Bioscience, Department of Biofunctional Chemistry, Graduate School of Natural Science and Technology, Okayama University, Japan

Kazuya Fukuoka and Takashi Nakano
Department of Respiratory Medicine, Hyogo College of Medicine, Japan

Takumi Kishimoto
Okayama Rosai Hospital, Japan

5. References

Asseman, C., Mauze, S., Leach, M.W., Coffman, R.L., & Powrie, F. (1999). An essential role for interleukin 10 in the function of regulatory T cells that inhibit intestinal inflammation. The Journal of experimental medicine, Vol.190, No.7, pp.995-1004, 0022-1007

Chen, X., Allan, D.S., Krzewski, K., Ge, B., Kopcow, H., & Strominger, J.L. (2006). CD28-stimulated ERK2 phosphorylation is required for polarization of the microtubule organizing center and granules in YTS NK cells. *Proc Natl Acad Sci U S A*, Vol.103, No.27, pp.10346-10351, ISSN 0027-8424

Chen, X., Trivedi, P.P., Ge, B., Krzewski, K., & Strominger, J.L. (2007). Many NK cell receptors activate ERK2 and JNK1 to trigger microtubule organizing center and granule polarization and cytotoxicity. *Proc Natl Acad Sci U S A*, Vol.104, No.15, pp.6329-6334, ISSN 0027-8424

Creaney, J., Van Bruggen, I., Hof, M., Segal, A., Musk, A.W., De Klerk, N., Horick, N., Skates, S.J., & Robinson, B.W. (2007). Combined CA125 and mesothelin levels for the diagnosis of malignant mesothelioma. *Chest*, Vol.132, No.4, pp.1239-1246, 0012-3692

Dieckmann, D., Bruett, C.H., Ploettner, H., Lutz, M.B., & Schuler, G. (2002). Human CD4(+)CD25(+) regulatory, contact-dependent T cells induce interleukin 10-producing, contact-independent type 1-like regulatory T cells [corrected]. The Journal of experimental medicine, Vol.196, No.2, pp.247-253, 0022-1007

Dodson, R.F., Williams, M.G., Jr., Corn, C.J., Brollo, A., & Bianchi, C. (1991). A comparison of asbestos burden in lung parenchyma, lymph nodes, and plaques. *Ann N Y Acad Sci*, Vol.643, pp.53-60, ISSN 0077-8923

Dufour, J.H., Dziejman, M., Liu, M.T., Leung, J.H., Lane, T.E., & Luster, A.D. (2002). IFN-gamma-inducible protein 10 (IP-10; CXCL10)-deficient mice reveal a role for IP-10 in effector T cell generation and trafficking. *J Immunol*, Vol.168, No.7, pp.3195-3204, ISSN 0022-1767

Dusinska, M., Collins, A., Kazimirova, A., Barancokova, M., Harrington, V., Volkovova, K., Staruchova, M., Horska, A., Wsolova, L., Kocan, A., Petrik, J., Machata, M., Ratcliffe, B., & Kyrtopoulos, S. (2004). Genotoxic effects of asbestos in humans. *Mutat Res*, Vol.553, No.1-2, pp.91-102, ISSN 0027-5107

Endt, J., Eissmann, P., Hoffmann, S.C., Meinke, S., Giese, T., & Watzl, C. (2007). Modulation of 2B4 (CD244) activity and regulated SAP expression in human NK cells. *Eur J Immunol*, Vol.37, No.1, pp.193-198, ISSN 0014-2980

Fontenot, J.D., & Rudensky, A.Y. (2005). A well adapted regulatory contrivance: regulatory T cell development and the forkhead family transcription factor Foxp3. *Nat Immunol*, Vol.6, No.4, pp.331-337, ISSN 1529-2908

Garni-Wagner, B.A., Purohit, A., Mathew, P.A., Bennett, M., & Kumar, V. (1993). A novel function-associated molecule related to non-MHC-restricted cytotoxicity mediated by activated natural killer cells and T cells. *J Immunol*, Vol.151, No.1, pp.60-70, ISSN 0022-1767

Gerber, B.O., Zanni, M.P., Uguccioni, M., Loetscher, M., Mackay, C.R., Pichler, W.J., Yawalkar, N., Baggiolini, M., & Moser, B. (1997). Functional expression of the eotaxin receptor CCR3 in T lymphocytes co-localizing with eosinophils. *Current biology : CB*, Vol.7, No.11, pp.836-843, ISSN 0960-9822

Green, E.A., Gorelik, L., Mcgregor, C.M., Tran, E.H., & Flavell, R.A. (2003). CD4+CD25+ T regulatory cells control anti-islet CD8+ T cells through TGF-beta-TGF-beta receptor interactions in type 1 diabetes. Proc Natl Acad Sci U S A, Vol.100, No.19, pp.10878-10883, 0027-8424

Homey, B., Muller, A., & Zlotnik, A. (2002). Chemokines: agents for the immunotherapy of cancer? Nat Rev Immunol, Vol.2, No.3, pp.175-184, 1474-1733

Imai, K., Matsuyama, S., Miyake, S., Suga, K., & Nakachi, K. (2000). Natural cytotoxic activity of peripheral-blood lymphocytes and cancer incidence: an 11-year follow-up study of a general population. *Lancet*, Vol.356, No.9244, pp.1795-1799, ISSN 0140-6736

Jonuleit, H., Schmitt, E., Kakirman, H., Stassen, M., Knop, J., & Enk, A.H. (2002). Infectious tolerance: human CD25(+) regulatory T cells convey suppressor activity to conventional CD4(+) T helper cells. The Journal of experimental medicine, Vol.196, No.2, pp.255-260, 0022-1007

Liew, F.Y. (2002). T(H)1 and T(H)2 cells: a historical perspective. *Nature reviews Immunology*, Vol.2, No.1, pp.55-60, ISSN 1474-1733

Luster, A.D., & Ravetch, J.V. (1987). Biochemical characterization of a gamma interferon-inducible cytokine (IP-10). The Journal of experimental medicine, Vol.166, No.4, pp.1084-1097, 0022-1007

Maeda, M., Nishimura, Y., Hayashi, H., Kumagai, N., Chen, Y., Murakami, S., Miura, Y., Hiratsuka, J.I., Kishimoto, T., & Otsuki, T. (2011). Reduction of CXCR3 in an in vitro Model of Continuous Asbestos Exposure on a Human T-cell Line, MT-2. *Am J Respir Cell Mol Biol*, Vo.45, No.3, pp.470-479, ISSN 1535-4989

Maeda, M., Nishimura, Y., Hayashi, H., Kumagai, N., Chen, Y., Murakami, S., Miura, Y., Hiratsuka, J.I., Kishimoto, T., & Otsuki, T. (2011). Decreased CXCR3 Expression in CD4+ T Cells Exposed to Asbestos or Derived from Asbestos-exposed Patients. *Am J Respir Cell Mol Biol*, Vo.45, No.4, pp.795-803, ISSN 1535-4989

Miserocchi, G., Sancini, G., Mantegazza, F., & Chiappino, G. (2008). Translocation pathways for inhaled asbestos fibers. *Environ Health*, Vol.7, pp.4, ISSN 1476-069X (Electronic)

Monney, L., Sabatos, C.A., Gaglia, J.L., Ryu, A., Waldner, H., Chernova, T., Manning, S., Greenfield, E.A., Coyle, A.J., Sobel, R.A., Freeman, G.J., & Kuchroo, V.K. (2002). Th1-specific cell surface protein Tim-3 regulates macrophage activation and severity of an autoimmune disease. *Nature*, Vol.415, No.6871, pp.536-541, ISSN 0028-0836

Moretta, A., Bottino, C., Vitale, M., Pende, D., Cantoni, C., Mingari, M.C., Biassoni, R., & Moretta, L. (2001). Activating receptors and coreceptors involved in human natural killer cell-mediated cytolysis. *Annu Rev Immunol*, Vol.19, pp.197-223, ISSN 0732-0582

Moretta, L., & Moretta, A. (2004). Unravelling natural killer cell function: triggering and inhibitory human NK receptors. *EMBO J*, Vol.23, No.2, pp.255-259, ISSN 0261-4189

Mossman, B.T., & Churg, A. (1998). Mechanisms in the pathogenesis of asbestosis and silicosis. *Am J Respir Crit Care Med*, Vol.157, No.5 Pt 1, pp.1666-1680, ISSN 1073-449X

Mossman, B.T., Kamp, D.W., & Weitzman, S.A. (1996). Mechanisms of carcinogenesis and clinical features of asbestos-associated cancers. *Cancer Invest*, Vol.14, No.5, pp.466-480, ISSN 0735-7907

Nishimura, Y., Maeda, M., Kumagai, N., Hayashi, H., Miura, Y., & Otsuki, T. (2009a). Decrease in phosphorylation of ERK following decreased expression of NK cell-activating receptors in human NK cell line exposed to asbestos. *Int J Immunopathol Pharmacol*, Vol.22, No.4, pp.879-888, ISSN 0394-6320

Nishimura, Y., Miura, Y., Maeda, M., Kumagai, N., Murakami, S., Hayashi, H., Fukuoka, K., Nakano, T., & Otsuki, T. (2009b). Impairment in cytotoxicity and expression of NK cell-activating receptors on human NK cells following exposure to asbestos fibers. *Int J Immunopathol Pharmacol*, Vol.22, No.3, pp.579-590, ISSN 0394-6320

Onda, M., Nagata, S., Ho, M., Bera, T.K., Hassan, R., Alexander, R.H., & Pastan, I. (2006). Megakaryocyte potentiation factor cleaved from mesothelin precursor is a useful tumor marker in the serum of patients with mesothelioma. Clinical cancer research : an official journal of the American Association for Cancer Research, Vol.12, No.14 Pt 1, pp.4225-4231, 1078-0432

Parker, D.C. (1993). T cell-dependent B cell activation. *Annu Rev Immunol*, Vol.11, pp.331-360, ISSN 0732-0582

Peck, A., & Mellins, E.D. (2009). Breaking old paradigms: Th17 cells in autoimmune arthritis. *Clin Immunol*, Vol.132, No.3, pp.295-304, ISSN 1521-7035

Qin, S., Rottman, J.B., Myers, P., Kassam, N., Weinblatt, M., Loetscher, M., Koch, A.E., Moser, B., & Mackay, C.R. (1998). The chemokine receptors CXCR3 and CCR5 mark subsets of T cells associated with certain inflammatory reactions. *The Journal of clinical investigation*, Vol.101, No.4, pp.746-754, ISSN 0021-9738

Sakaguchi, S. (2005). Naturally arising Foxp3-expressing CD25+CD4+ regulatory T cells in immunological tolerance to self and non-self. *Nat Immunol*, Vol.6, No.4, pp.345-352, ISSN 1529-2908

Sallusto, F., & Lanzavecchia, A. (2000). Understanding dendritic cell and T-lymphocyte traffic through the analysis of chemokine receptor expression. *Immunol Rev*, Vol.177, pp.134-140, ISSN 0105-2896

Sivori, S., Pende, D., Bottino, C., Marcenaro, E., Pessino, A., Biassoni, R., Moretta, L., & Moretta, A. (1999). NKp46 is the major triggering receptor involved in the natural cytotoxicity of fresh or cultured human NK cells. Correlation between surface density of NKp46 and natural cytotoxicity against autologous, allogeneic or xenogeneic target cells. *Eur J Immunol*, Vol.29, No.5, pp.1656-1666, ISSN 0014-2980

Smith, C.M., Wilson, N.S., Waithman, J., Villadangos, J.A., Carbone, F.R., Heath, W.R., & Belz, G.T. (2004). Cognate CD4(+) T cell licensing of dendritic cells in CD8(+) T cell immunity. *Nat Immunol*, Vol.5, No.11, pp.1143-1148, ISSN 1529-2908

Smyth, M.J., Cretney, E., Takeda, K., Wiltrout, R.H., Sedger, L.M., Kayagaki, N., Yagita, H., & Okumura, K. (2001). Tumor necrosis factor-related apoptosis-inducing ligand (TRAIL) contributes to interferon gamma-dependent natural killer cell protection from tumor metastasis. *The Journal of experimental medicine*, Vol.193, No.6, pp.661-670, ISSN 0022-1007

Sporn, T.A., & Roggli, V.L. (2004) Mesothelioma. In: *Pathology of Asbestos-Associated Diseases*, V.L. Roggli, T.D. Oury, T.A. Sporn, pp.104-168, Springer-Verlag, ISBN 978-1441918949, New York

Takeda, K., Hayakawa, Y., Smyth, M.J., Kayagaki, N., Yamaguchi, N., Kakuta, S., Iwakura, Y., Yagita, H., & Okumura, K. (2001). Involvement of tumor necrosis factor-related apoptosis-inducing ligand in surveillance of tumor metastasis by liver natural killer cells. *Nat Med*, Vol.7, No.1, pp.94-100, ISSN 1078-8956

Topinka, J., Loli, P., Georgiadis, P., Dusinska, M., Hurbankova, M., Kovacikova, Z., Volkovova, K., Kazimirova, A., Barancokova, M., Tatrai, E., Oesterle, D., Wolff, T., & Kyrtopoulos, S.A. (2004). Mutagenesis by asbestos in the lung of lambda-lacI transgenic rats. *Mutat Res*, Vol.553, No.1-2, pp.67-78, ISSN 0027-5107

Trapani, J.A., & Smyth, M.J. (2002). Functional significance of the perforin/granzyme cell death pathway. *Nat Rev Immunol*, Vol.2, No.10, pp.735-747, ISSN 1474-1733

Valiante, N.M., & Trinchieri, G. (1993). Identification of a novel signal transduction surface molecule on human cytotoxic lymphocytes. *J Exp Med*, Vol.178, No.4, pp.1397-1406, ISSN 0022-1007

Vivier, E., Tomasello, E., Baratin, M., Walzer, T., & Ugolini, S. (2008). Functions of natural killer cells. *Nat Immunol*, Vol.9, No.5, pp.503-510, ISSN 1529-2916

Wendel, M., Galani, I.E., Suri-Payer, E., & Cerwenka, A. (2008). Natural killer cell accumulation in tumors is dependent on IFN-gamma and CXCR3 ligands. *Cancer Res*, Vol.68, No.20, pp.8437-8445, ISSN 1538-7445

Yokoyama, W.M., & Plougastel, B.F. (2003). Immune functions encoded by the natural killer gene complex. *Nat Rev Immunol*, Vol.3, No.4, pp.304-316, ISSN 1474-1733

Chapter 3

Role of Inflammation and Angiogenic Growth Factors in Malignant Mesothelioma

Loredana Albonici, Camilla Palumbo and Vittorio Manzari

Additional information is available at the end of the chapter

http://dx.doi.org/10.5772/47951

1. Introduction

Malignant mesothelioma (MM) is a highly aggressive tumor which arises from the mesothelial cell lining of the serosal surfaces, most cases (>90%) being of pleural origin (Attanoos & Gibbs, 1997; Robinson & Lake, 2005). The pathogenesis of MM has been mainly associated with previous asbestos exposure (Berman & Crump, 2008), with a latency period of up to 40 years, although other agents such as Simian virus 40 (SV40) or genetic susceptibility factors have been linked to the development of this tumor (Carbone et al., 2002; Pisick & Salgia, 2005). Indeed, human mesothelial cells are highly susceptible to SV40-mediated transformation *in vitro* and SV40 DNA sequences and large T antigen (Tag) have been detected in human MM cells (Bocchetta et al., 2000; Carbone et al., 2012; Gazdar et al., 2003).

MM is largely unresponsive to conventional chemotherapy or radiotherapy and, despite its low metastatic efficiency, it is highly invasive to surrounding tissues so that its extensive growth leads to the failure of the organs underlying the serosal membranes (Astoul, 1999). In fact, the primary cause of fatality in MM is related to the propensity of the tumor cells to invade locally, even though MM metastasis are more common after surgery and, at the autopsy, metastatic diffusion is observed in 50% of patients (Astoul, 1999). At present, the median survival from diagnosis of MM is less than two years (Palumbo et al., 2008).

The mesothelium is not just a passive protective surface, but a highly dynamic membrane (Mutsaers, 2004). It consists of a single layer of elongated, flattened, squamous-like cells of mesodermal origin, characterized by dual epithelial/mesenchymal features. Cuboidal mesothelial cells can also be found at various locations in physiological conditions. Further, mesothelial cells can adopt a cuboidal morphology, which reflects a metabolically activated state, after injury or stimulation of the serosal surface (Mutsaers, 2004). Indeed, mesothelial cells are sentinel cells that can sense and respond to a variety of signals within their microenvironment. They participate in serosal inflammation by secreting both pro- and anti-inflammatory as well as immunomodulatory mediators. Besides, these cells can act as antigen presenting cells for T lymphocytes (Hausmann et al., 2000), regulate tissue repair, control fibrin deposition and breakdown, and modulate adhesion, growth and dissemination of tumor cells metastasizing to the serosal membranes (Mutsaers, 2002). In particular, in response to different types of stimuli, including cytokines and asbestos fibers, mesothelial cells have been reported to release prostaglandins, chemokines, reactive oxygen and nitrogen species and growth factors which represent key effectors in the modulation of inflammatory reactions that occur in response to pleural injury (Fleury-Feith et al., 2003; Mutsaers, 2002).

2. Asbestos-induced carcinogenesis as an inflammation-driven process

The association between exposure to asbestos fibers and development of lung cancer and mesothelioma is well established in both humans and animals models (Greillier & Astoul, 2008; Huang et al., 2011; Mossman & Churg, 1998; Yarborough, 2007). A variety of mediators, either generated directly from asbestos fibers or elaborated intracellularly or extracellularly by cells exposed to asbestos, are implicated in the initiation and promotion of mesothelial cell transformation.

The mechanisms underlying asbestos-induced carcinogenesis involve mutagenic and non-mutagenic pathways, the latter including inflammation, enhanced mitogenesis, cell signaling alterations, and cytotoxic apoptosis/necrosis. Neither of these two mechanisms alone fully accounts for the complex biological abnormalities produced by asbestos fibers, even though in MM asbestos appears to act as a complete carcinogen (Dong et al., 1994; Huang et al., 2011). Still, the chronic inflammatory response induced by asbestos inhalation seems to play a critical role in mesothelial cell transformation.

Asbestos exposure induces an inflammatory reaction with a large component of mononuclear phagocytes (Antony et al., 1993; Branchaud et al., 1993; Carbone et al., 2012; Choe et al., 1997). Upon differentiation into macrophages, these cells phagocytize asbestos fibers and, in response, release numerous cytokines and reactive oxygen species with mutagenic properties (Robledo & Mossman, 1999). Thus, many of the pathological consequences occurring in the lung following exposure to asbestos fibers are believed to arise from an inflammatory cascade involving both autocrine and paracrine events (Hillegass et al., 2010). Persistent pulmonary inflammation is observed in animal models of asbestosis that can be correlated with fibroproliferative responses (Mossman & Churg, 1998).

Experimental models, as well as *in vitro* studies, have shown that mesothelial cells are particularly susceptible to the cytotoxic effects of asbestos (Baldys et al., 2007; BéruBé et al., 1996; Broaddus et al., 1996). Asbestos does not induce transformation of primary human mesothelial cells *in vitro*, instead, it is very cytotoxic to this cell type, causing extensive cell death. This finding raised an apparent paradoxical issue of how asbestos causes MM if human mesothelial cells exposed to this mineral die (Liu et al., 2000). This apparent paradox is reconciled by the current hypothesis that the chronic inflammation induced by asbestos leads to the persistent activation of the nuclear factor kappa B (NF-κB) transcription factor, which in turn mediates the activation of prosurvival genes and prevents apoptosis of the damaged mesothelial cells (Mantovani et al., 2008; Micheau & Tschopp, 2003; Philip et al., 2004). This allows mesothelial cells with asbestos-induced DNA damage to survive and divide rather than die and, if sufficient genetic damage accumulates, to eventually develop into a MM (Miura et al., 2006; Nymark, 2007). In fact, apoptosis is an important mechanism by which cells with DNA damage are eliminated without eliciting an inflammatory response (Ullrich et al., 2008; Yoshida et al., 2010). However, failure of apoptosis in cells with unrepaired DNA and chromosomal damage after chronic exposure to asbestos may lead to permanent genetic alterations and trigger the development of a clone of cancerous cells (Roos & Kaina, 2006; Wu, 2006). Consistently, MM cells are found to be apoptosis-resistant as compared to primary cultured mesothelial cells (Fennel & Rudd, 2004; Villanova et al., 2008).

2.1. Tumor Necrosis Factor-α and other pro-inflammatory cytokines

Tumor Necrosis Factor-α (TNF-α) is probably the most studied candidate for initiating inflammatory and fibrotic events linked to lung diseases such as asbestosis. Asbestos fibers cause the accumulation of macrophages in the pleura and lung. When these macrophages encounter asbestos, they release TNF-α. At the same time, asbestos induces the secretion of TNF-α and the expression of TNF-α receptor I (TNF-RI) in mesothelial cells (Yang et al., 2006). Remarkably, treatment of mesothelial cells with TNF-α significantly reduced asbestos cytotoxicity. Indeed, TNF-α activates NF-κB, which in turn promotes mesothelial cell survival and resistance to the cytotoxic effects of asbestos. Thus, TNF-α signaling through NF-κB-dependent mechanisms increases the percentage of mesothelial cells that survive asbestos exposure, thereby increasing the pool of asbestos-damaged cells susceptible to malignant transformation (Haegens et al., 2007; Janssen-Heininger et al., 1999; Yang et al., 2006).

It has been reported that rats receiving a single intratracheal instillation of fibrogenic chrysotile asbestos developed lung chronic inflammatory reactions characterized by the accumulation of alveolar macrophages producing elevated levels of both Interleukin (IL)-1 and IL-6 (Lemaire & Ouellet, 1996). An increased production and/or release of these cytokines triggers inflammatory cell recruitment, thus amplifying and sustaining local inflammation. It has also been demonstrated that crocidolite asbestos and TNF-α can stimulate a dose-dependent increase in IL-6 expression and secretion from cultured, transformed and normal, human alveolar type II epithelial cells that is dependent upon intracellular redox potential (Simeonova et al., 1997). Interestingly, although MM cells appear to express low levels of IL-6 receptor (IL-6R), IL-6 can act as a growth factor for these cells through a trans-signaling mechanism involving the interaction of macromolecular complexes of IL-6 and soluble IL-6R (sIL-6R) with the transmembrane glycoprotein gp130 expressed on the surface of MM cells (Adachi et al., 2006; Rose-John et al., 2007). High levels of both IL-6 and sIL-6R are typical of several chronic inflammatory conditions (Rose-John et al., 2007).

Thus, inflammatory cytokines such as TNF-α and IL-6 appear to play a dual role in MM pathogenesis: they induce and sustain pleural inflammation and at the same time can act as survival or mitogenic factors for normal and transformed mesothelial cells, respectively.

2.2. Reactive Oxygen and Nitrogen Species (ROS/RNS)

The mechanisms of injury and disease development caused by asbestos fibers are presumed to be related to their greater fibrogenic and carcinogenic properties in comparison to other minerals. Asbestos–induced mutagenicity is mediated through both direct and indirect pathways. Asbestos fibers may induce mutagenicity and genotoxicity directly through physical interaction with the mitotic machinery after being phagocytized by the target cells, or indirectly as a result of DNA and chromosome damage caused by asbestos-induced reactive oxygen (ROS) and nitrogen species (RNS) (Kamp & Weitzman, 1999; Shukla et al., 2003a, 2003b). ROS and RNS can be generated primarily by asbestos fibers or secondarily through fiber-induced inflammation (Aust et al., 2011; Gulumian, 2005; Hoidal, 2001). Free radicals generated from asbestos fibers plus the direct damage induced by the fibers are linked to cell signaling, inflammation, and a plethora of other responses (mutagenesis, proliferation, etc.) associated with the pathogenesis of asbestos-associated diseases (Heinz et al., 2010; Manning et al., 2002; Shukla et al., 2003a, 2003b).

Several evidences indicate that a main factor in determining the surface and biological reactivity of different types of asbestos fibers is their ability to participate in redox reactions that generate free radicals (Kamp & Weitzman, 1999; Shukla et al., 2003a). Although the nature of the free radical-generating surface sites on asbestos fibers is not yet clear, asbestos fibers have an intrinsic redox activity and contain ferrous iron, which catalyzes reactions generating active oxygen intermediates on the fiber surface. Within the tissues several asbestos fiber types can produce reactive oxygen free radicals from hydrogen peroxide, a common product of intermediary tissue metabolism. Epidemiological studies have identified crocidolite as one of the most potent forms of asbestos associated with the induction of MM (Heintz et al., 2010). Crocidolite has a greater surface-area and a higher ferrous iron content compared to other fiber types such as chrysotile, and it is more biologically active in the generation of free radicals (Toyokuni, 2009). However, the ability of asbestos fibers to elicit these effects is not related to total iron content, suggesting the presence of specific iron active sites at the fibers' surface (Shukla et al., 2003a).

Cells exposed to asbestos have also been reported to produce a higher amount of nitric oxide (NO). In this regard, it has been reported that in human mesothelial cells crocidolite increases the expression of the inducible NO synthase (NOS) isoform (iNOS), the activity of the constitutive endothelial NOS (eNOS), and the synthesis of NO via NF-κB and Akt activation (Riganti et al., 2007). Thus, the asbestos-induced upregulation of iNOS or NO in the lungs, as well as the induction of inflammation by fibers, may contribute along with ROS, to the pathogenesis of lung and pleural injury (Hussain et al., 2003; Tanaka et al., 1998). Indeed, ROS and RNS can cause breakage of DNA, lipid peroxidation, release of inflammatory cytokines such as TNF-α, and the modification of cellular proteins including phosphatases involved in cell signaling cascades (Gossart et al., 1996; Hussain et al., 2003), so that their increased synthesis by various cell types may have multiple roles in cellular events critical to the establishment of lung and pleural inflammation and uncontrolled cell proliferation.

Finally, in mesothelial and lung epithelial cells asbestos fibers, as opposed to nonpathogenic minerals, cause a persistent induction of the redox-sensitive transcription factors NF-κB and Activator Protein-1 (AP-1), which is accompanied by chronic alterations in gene expression (Heintz et al., 1993; Janssen et al., 1995). As mentioned above, the aberrant activation of the NF-κB pathway is regarded as a critical event for mesothelial cell transformation (Toyooka et al., 2008).

2.3. Transcription factors

2.3.1. NF-κB

NF-κB proteins are dimeric transcription factors composed of five different subunits, namely p65 (RelA), RelB, c-Rel, NF-κB1 p50 and NF-κB2 p52, which regulate gene expression events that impact on cell survival and differentiation. Moreover, since activation of NF-κB is critical in up-regulating the expression of many genes linked to proliferation, apoptosis resistance, and chemokine/cytokine production, this is undoubtedly a critical transcription factor in inflammatory responses occurring in target cells of asbestos-related diseases (Janssen et al., 1995, 1997).

In unstimulated cells, the NF-κB transcription dimers are retained in the cytoplasm in an inactive state through the interaction with a family of inhibitors called IκBs (Inhibitors of κB) or with the p50 and p52 precursor proteins, p105 and p100, respectively (Hayden & Ghosh, 2008; Scheidereit, 2006). Indeed, p50 and p52 are translated as precursors proteins containing an IκB-like C-terminal portion (Sun, 2011).

Two different NF-κB-activation pathways exist: the classical and the alternative NF-κB pathway. The classical NF-κB pathway is initiated by signals elicited by diverse receptors, including TNF receptors type 1/2, Toll/IL-1 receptor, T-cell and B-cell receptors and EGF receptor, and also by cellular stresses and DNA damage (Hayden & Ghosh 2004; Le Page et al., 2005). These signals induce the activation of the IκB kinase (IKK) complex, which is composed by the catalytic subunits IKKα and IKKβ and by the regulatory subunit IKKγ/NEMO (Hayden & Ghosh, 2008; Scheidereit, 2006; Sun, 2011). The activated IKK complex phosphorylates IκB proteins, thereby triggering their proteasomal degradation. As a consequence, NF-κB dimers are released and can translocate into the nucleus. This pathway mainly leads to the activation of p50:RelA dimers (Sun, 2011). Conversely, the alternative NF-κB pathway predominantly targets activation of RelB:p52 complexes. This pathway relies on the inducible processing of p100 triggered by signaling from TNF receptor family members via the NF-κB-inducing kinase (NIK): NIK activates IKKα, which, in turn, phosphorylates p100 and triggers its processing to p52. This event results in the conversion of p100-inhibited NF-κB complexes into p52-containing NF-κB dimers, capable of translocating into the nucleus (Hayden & Ghosh, 2008; Scheidereit, 2006; Sun, 2011).

NF-κB-regulated genes have distinct requirements for NF-κB dimers. For instance, the NF-κB binding site of the IL-2 gene has been reported to bind preferentially c-Rel homodimers and p50:c-Rel, while that of the gene encoding IL-8 has been found to selectively bind Rel A (Hoffman et al., 2003, 2006). On the other hand, several genes are redundantly induced by more than one dimer (Hoffman et al., 2003, 2006; Saccani et al., 2003).

A number of studies have shown that nuclear retention and DNA binding of NF-κB protein complexes are increased following exposure of various cell types to a variety of extracellular stimuli that include oxidative stress (Bowie & O'Neill, 2000), hypoxia (Jung et al., 2003; Royds et al., 1998) and inflammatory cytokines (Mantovani et al., 2008). These observations are consistent with the hypothesis that persistent activation of NF-κB can contribute to the induction of multiple genes that are critical to the pathogenesis of asbestos-associated diseases, since oxidants, local hypoxia and inflammatory cytokines are all components involved in the effects induced by asbestos exposure.

It is noteworthy that among various carcinogenic and non-carcinogenic fibers studied for their effect on nuclear translocation of NF-κB, only carcinogenic fibers were found to cause a dose-dependent translocation of this transcription factor to the nucleus, and this effect was reported to be oxidative stress-dependent (Brown et al., 1999). In lung macrophages, the asbestos-induced expression and secretion of TNF-α are mediated by iron-catalyzed ROS products (Simeonova & Luster, 1995) through a process that involves NF-κB activation (Cheng et al., 1999). In rat alveolar type 2 cells, the crocidolite-induced activation of NF-κB as well as the expression of the macrophage inflammatory protein-2 (MIP-2) gene have also been shown to be dependent on mitochondrial-derived oxidative stress (Driscoll et al., 1998).

2.3.2. *AP-1*

AP-1 is a homo- or heterodimeric transcription factor composed by proteins encoded by the *fos* and *jun* early response proto-oncogenes. This family of proteins includes c-Fos, FosB, FosL1 (Fra-1), FosL2 (Fra-2), c-Jun, JunB and JunD (Milde-Langosch, 2005). Whereas Jun members are capable of forming homodimers able to bind DNA and regulate transcription, all Fos members must form heterodimers with Jun family members to bind DNA.

AP-1 is a redox-sensitive transcription factor typically associated with cell proliferation and tumor promotion (Eferl & Wagner, 2003). The first evidence showing that asbestos exerts regulatory effects linked to aberrant transcriptional responses, cell proliferation and cell transformation derives from studies in which asbestos fibers caused induction of *c-fos* and *c-jun* proto-oncogene mRNAs in pleural mesothelial cells and tracheo-bronchial epithelial cells in a dose–response fashion (Heintz et al., 1993).

The persistent induction of AP-1 by asbestos suggests a model of asbestos-induced carcinogenesis involving chronic stimulation of cell proliferation through activation of early response genes (Schonthaler et al., 2011). Of note, early response genes are a set of genes whose transcription is rapidly induced in response to growth factors. Furthermore, AP-1 activity is induced by growth factors, pro-inflammatory cytokines and genotoxic stress (Jochum et al., 2001; Shaulian & Karin, 2002). These stimuli activate mitogen-activated protein kinase (MAPK) cascades through the phosphorylation of distinct substrates such as

ERK, JNK and p38 MAPK (Chang & Karin, 2001). Indeed, the MAPK signal transduction pathway uses AP-1 as a converging point not only to regulate the expression of various genes but also to autoregulate AP-1 gene transcription (Reuter et al., 2010).

Several genes, which play very important roles in injury, repair, and differentiation, contain binding site(s) for AP-1 in their promoter and/or enhancer regions (Chang & Karin, 2001). These genes include extracellular matrix metalloproteinases (MMPs), antioxidant enzymes, growth factors and their receptors, differentiation markers, cytokines, chemokines and other transcription factors (Shaulian & Karin, 2001).

2.3.3. Nuclear Factor of Activated T Cells (NFAT)

The Nuclear Factor of Activated T cells (NFAT) family of transcription factors consists of five proteins that are evolutionarily related to the Rel/NF-κB family. NFAT can be present in both the cytoplasm and the nucleus. In the cytoplasm NFAT is in a highly phosphorylated, inactive state. Cell stimuli leading to the elevation of intracellular Ca^{2+} levels induce the activation of the phosphatase PP2B/Calcineurin which dephosphorylates NFAT. This results in its nuclear relocalization and transcriptional activation. Interestingly, NFAT family members can act synergistically with AP-1 on composite DNA elements which contain adjacent NFAT and AP-1 binding sites (Macián et al., 2001). A functional cooperation has also been reported to occur between NFAT and NF-κB (Jash et al., 2012).

Initially, NFAT was identified in lymphocytes and was reported to be expressed in activated but not resting T cells (Macián et al., 2005; Shaw et al., 1988). NFAT regulates not only T cell activation and differentiation but also the function of other immune cells, including dendritic cells (DCs), B cells and megakaryocytes. In addition, NFAT has crucial roles in numerous developmental programs in vertebrates.

Dysregulation of NFAT signalling is now known to be associated with malignant transformation and the development of cancer (Mancini & Toker, 2009; Müller & Rao, 2010). The observation that NFAT can be activated by asbestos-induced oxidative stress suggests that this transcription factor may play multiple roles in asbestos-induced inflammation and carcinogenesis (Li et al., 2002). Indeed, NFAT mediates the expression of several inflammatory cytokines, including TNF-α, and is involved in cell transformation, proliferation, invasive migration, tumor cell survival and tumor angiogenesis (Mancini & Toker, 2009).

3. Multifaceted role of angiogenic growth factors in MM

Angiogenesis is a common feature of solid tumors. Indeed, the development of a clinically observable tumor requires the neoformation of a vascular network sufficient to sustain tumor growth (Ribatti et al., 2007). Tumor angiogenesis is stimulated by the secretion of angiogenic molecules which induce endothelial cells from nearby vessels to switch from a quiescent to an activated state. Further, upon the stimulation of angiogenic growth factors, activated endothelial cells disrupt the extracellular matrix, proliferate and migrate (Ribatti et al., 2007). Angiogenic growth factors include, among the others, Vascular Endothelial Growth Factor (VEGF), Placenta Growth Factor (PlGF), Platelet-Derived Growth Factor (PDGF) and acidic and basic Fibroblast Growth Factors (FGF-1 and -2, respectively). VEGF is regarded as the most important player in angiogenesis (Ono, 2008).

The link between angiogenesis and tumor progression is provided by the negative prognostic value of intratumoral microvascular density (IMD) (Folkman, 2006; Kerbel, 2008). In MM the IMD has an independent prognostic value (Kumar-Singh et al., 1997). MM demonstrates a higher IMD than colon and breast tumors and, consistently, presents with minimal central necrosis despite its huge size (Gasparini & Harris, 1995; Kumar-Singh et al., 1997).

On the other hand, the involvement of angiogenic growth factors in MM goes beyond the stimulation of angiogenesis. Indeed, as discussed below, MM cells express receptors for several angiogenic factors which, accordingly, can directly modulate MM cell behavior.

3.1. Angiogenic growth factors of the VEGF family

The human VEGF family consists of five members: VEGF (VEGF-A), VEGF-B, VEGF-C, VEGF-D and PlGF. These growth factors are secreted as dimers and their biological effects are mediated by binding to three tyrosine kinase receptors, *i.e.* VEGF-R1/Flt-1, VEGF-R2/KDR (whose murine homologue is known as Flk-1) and VEGF-R3/Flt-4, and two non-enzymatic co-receptors known as neuropilin-1 and -2 (Ferrara et al., 2003; Koch et al., 2011; Roskoski, 2007).

3.1.1. VEGF

VEGF is regarded as the major mediator of tumor angiogenesis. It is expressed in the majority of cancers and has a central role in tumor growth and metastasis. In fact, this growth factor is essential for the mobilization of bone-marrow-derived endothelial precursors in neovascularization (Asahara et al., 1999), and stimulates vascular endothelial cells mobility, proliferation and survival (Waltenberger et al., 1994).

High levels of VEGF are present both in malignant and non-malignant pleural effusions leading to increased vascular permeability. On the other hand, VEGF levels in serum or pleural effusions of MM patients are higher than those found in patients with non-malignant pleuritis or lung cancer involving malignant pleural effusions. Further, in MM patients elevated serum or pleural effusion levels of VEGF correlate with a worse prognosis and may also contribute to increase resistance to chemotherapy (Hirayama et al., 2011; Yasumitsu et al., 2010; Zebrowski et al., 1999). In fact, VEGF status has proved to be of value in predicting the effectiveness of radiotherapy and chemotherapy on different cancers (Choi et al., 2008; Kumar et al., 2009; Toi et al., 2001).

In addition to its role in tumor vascularization, VEGF can directly affect the behavior of cancer cells in an autocrine or paracrine manner. Indeed, many tumor cell types express VEGF receptors. VEGF has been found to promote the growth of transformed cell lines *in vitro* (Masood et al., 2001) and to act as a survival factor for tumor cells by enhancing the expression of the antiapoptotic factors bcl-2 (Harmey & Bouchier-Hayes, 2002) and survivin (Kanwar et al., 2011). In this context, MM cells have been shown to express high amounts of VEGF, VEGF receptors and co-receptors both *in vitro* and *in vivo*, and VEGF has been demonstrated to act as an autocrine growth factor for this tumor cell type (Albonici et al., 2009; Ohta et al., 1999; Pompeo et al., 2009; Strizzi et al., 2001a).

VEGF-R1 participates in cell migration; it has an important role in monocyte chemotaxis and promotes recruitment of circulating endothelial precursor cells from bone marrow (Hattori et al., 2002). Its expression is increased in various tumors, correlates with disease progression and can predict poor prognosis, metastasis and recurrent disease in humans (Dawson et al., 2009; Fischer et al., 2008; Kerber et al., 2008). This receptor is also expressed by MM cells *in vitro* and *in vivo*, where it appears to mediate proliferative and cell survival responses (Albonici et al., 2009; Strizzi et al., 2001a).

VEGF-R2 is the main mediator of VEGF-stimulated endothelial cell migration, proliferation, survival and enhanced vascular permeability (Olsson et al., 2006; Shibuya, 2006). VEGF-R2 expression is induced in conjunction with active angiogenesis, such as during the reparative process, and in pathological conditions associated with neovascularization, such as cancer (Plate et al., 1993). VEGF-R2 is overexpressed in MM cells and specimens, and VEGF-R2 silencing by small intefering RNA has been shown to induce cell death in MM or immortalized mesotelial cells *in vitro* (Albonici et al., 2009; Catalano et al., 2009; Pompeo et al., 2009; Strizzi et al., 2001a). Interestingly, it has been reported that in MM cells this receptor can be activated also via the semaphorin-6D receptor Plexin-A1, triggering a prosurvival program that promotes anchorage-independent growth through a NF-κB-dependent pathway (Catalano et al., 2009). Remarkably, the expression of plexin-A1 is induced by asbestos fibers and overexpression of plexin-A1 in non-malignant mesothelial cells inhibits cell death after asbestos exposure, thus suggesting a role for this receptor not only in MM promotion and progression but also in asbestos-induced mesothelial carcinogenesis (Catalano et al., 2009).

In vitro studies have shown that transfection of normal mesothelial cells with SV40 Tag potently increases VEGF protein and mRNA levels (Cacciotti et al., 2002) as well as mesothelial cell proliferation (Catalano et al., 2002). These data indicate that VEGF regulation by SV40 transforming proteins can also represent a key event in MM onset and progression.

3.1.2. PlGF

PlGF, originally identified in the placenta during the early embryonic development (Khaliq et al., 1996; Maglione et al., 1991), is expressed in several other organs including the heart, lung, thyroid, skeletal muscle and adipose tissue (Persico et al., 1999) but not normal mesothelium (Albonici et al., 2009).

Although the role exerted by PlGF in tumor growth is controversial yet, PlGF can stimulate vessel growth and maturation directly by affecting endothelial and mural cells, as well as indirectly by recruiting pro-angiogenic cell types (Barillari et al., 1998; Carmeliet, 2003). It also promotes the recruitment and maturation of angiogenesis-competent myeloid progenitors to growing sprouts and collateral vessels (Hattori et al., 2002; Luttun et al., 2002; Rafii et al., 2003). Further, PlGF is able to protect endothelial cells from apoptosis, in a similar manner as VEGF, by inducing the expression of antiapoptotic genes such as survivin (Adini et al., 2002).

Under pathological conditions, PlGF abundance is elevated in various cell types and tissues, including vascular endothelial cells, and many different tumor cells (Albonici et al., 2009; Cao et al., 1996; Fischer et al., 2007; Oura et al., 2003). PlGF expression is switched on in hyperplastic/reactive mesothelium and in MM cells (Albonici et al., 2009). Moreover, in MM as well as in different types of cancer, including melanoma, gastric, colorectal and breast carcinomas, PlGF plasma levels and intratumoral expression have been found to correlate with tumor stage, vascularity, recurrence, metastasis and survival (Chen et al., 2004; Marcellini et al., 2006; Parr et al. 2005; Pompeo et al.; 2009; Wei et al., 2005).

In vitro studies have shown that administration of recombinant PlGF to MM cells triggers the activation of Akt but does not elicit a significant stimulation of cell growth. Conversely, the administration of PlGF-neutralizing antibodies causes a significant reduction of MM cell viability, demonstrating the PlGF acts as a survival factor for MM cells (Albonici et al., 2009).

PlGF binds VEGF-R1 and the co-receptors neuropilin-1 and -2, but, unlike VEGF, it does not bind VEGF-R2. Accordingly, it can act independently of VEGF in cells which primarily express VEGF-R1 (Fischer et al., 2007). Worthy of note, even though VEGF and PlGF both bind VEGF-R1, PlGF was reported to stimulate the phosphorylation of specific VEGF-R1 tyrosine residues and the expression of distinct downstream target genes as compared to VEGF (Autiero et al., 2003). On the other hand, PlGF can also sustain VEGF activity through different mechanisms involving both VEGF-R1 and VEGF-R2. One of these mechanisms relies on the formation of PlGF:VEGF heterodimers. Indeed, PlGF:VEGF heterodimers have been isolated from cells producing both factors and shown to bind VEGF-R1:VEGF-R2 receptor complexes, thus inducing receptor cross-talk and activation of VEGF-R2, the major mediator of VEGF activities (Autiero et al., 2003; Cao et al., 1996). In addition, the activation of VEGF-R1 by PlGF homodimers may induce the intermolecular transphosphorylation and activation of VEGF-R2 (Carmeliet et al., 2001).

It is noteworthy that *in vivo* anti-PlGF treatment was reported to inhibit tumor growth without affecting healthy vessels, thus reducing tumor infiltration by angiogenic macrophages and severe tumor hypoxia, and preventing the switch on of the angiogenic rescue program leading to the enhanced release different angiogenic factors responsible for resistance to VEGF receptors inhibitors (Fischer et al., 2007).

3.2. PDGF

PDGFs comprise a family of dimeric growth factors structurally and functionally related to VEGFs (Andrae et al., 2008). PDGF homodimers are formed by four different chains, *i.e.* PDGF-A, PDGF-B, PDGF-C and PDGF-D. In addition, PDGF-A and –B chains can form the heterodimeric PDGF-AB. The biological effects of PDGF are mediated by two tyrosine kinase receptors, namely the PDGF receptor alpha (PDGFRα), which binds PDGF-A, -B, and –C chains, and the PDGF receptor beta (PDGFR), which binds PDGF-B and –D. Accordingly, upon ligand binding different receptor dimers may form depending on ligand configuration and the pattern of receptor expression. Cellular responses to PDGF signaling include stimulation of cell growth, differentiation, migration and inhibition of apoptosis (Andrae et al., 2008).

An increased PDGF activity has been linked with tumors, vascular and fibrotic diseases (Andrae et al., 2008). Autocrine PDGF signaling leading to enhanced proliferation of tumor cells occurs in several types of cancer (Ostman, 2004). In addition, PDGF secretion by cancer cells and activated endothelial cells promotes the formation of both fibrous and vascular tumor stroma. In particular, PDGF-BB participates in tumor angiogenesis by stimulating endothelial cell motility and pericyte recruitment to neoformed vessels, thus leading to vessel stabilization, tumor cell survival and growth. Instead, both PDGF-AA and PDGF-BB appear involved in tumor recruitment of PDGFR-positive fibroblasts which, in turn, can be activated by PDGFs to produce VEGF and other tumor-promoting growth factors (Andrae et al., 2008; Cao et al., 2008; Homsi & Daud, 2007).

Either high PDGF-AB serum levels or a strong expression of PDGFR signaling effectors in MM tissues have been associated with a lower survival in MM patients (Filiberti et al., 2005; Kothmaier et al., 2008). In fact, several evidence support a role for PDGF in MM promotion and progression through both autocrine and paracrine mechanisms.

While PDGFRα expression levels are lower in MM than in normal mesothelial cells, PDGFRβ, PDGF-A and PDGF-B are overexpressed in MM cells as compared to their non-transformed counterparts (Langerak et al., 1996a, 1996b; Metheny-Barlow et al., 2001). Functional studies have shown that transduction of MM cells with a hammerhead ribozyme against PDGFRβ mRNA reduced both PDGFRβ expression and MM cell proliferation, demonstrating the involvement of a PDGF-BB autocrine loop in MM cell growth (Dorai et al., 1994). Conversely, the role of PDGF-A in MM cell proliferation is controversial. Indeed, the transfection of MM cells with antisense oligonucleotides to PDGF-A has been reported to either inhibit or stimulate MM cell growth *in vitro* (Garlepp & Leong, 1995; Metheny-Barlow et al., 2001). On the other hand, PDGF-A appears to play an important role in sustaining MM cell growth *in vivo* through paracrine mechanisms. Indeed, PDGF-A overexpression in MM cells inoculated in nude mice was found to increase tumor incidence, tumor growth rate and to decrease the latency period to tumor formation (Metheny-Barlow et al., 2001). In this regard, it has been suggested that PDGF-A participates in a malignant cytokine network through which MM cells instigates tumor-associated fibroblasts to produce growth factors, such as hepatocyte growth factor (HGF), with tumor-promoting activities (Li et al., 2011).

3.3. FGF

The FGF family encompasses 22 structurally related ligands in mammals. The effects of most FGF family members, including FGF-1 and -2, are mediated by binding to a family of tyrosine kinase receptors designated FGF receptors (FGFR1 to FGFR5), whereas a smaller number of FGF isoforms does not bind FGFRs but interacts with voltage-gated sodium channels (Knights & Cook, 2010).

FGFs regulate cell proliferation, differentiation, survival, wound healing and angiogenesis. In cancer, FGF signaling is frequently de-regulated, resulting in mitogenic, anti-apoptotic and angiogenic responses (Knights & Cook, 2010). FGF-1 and -2, but also other less-studied FGF isoforms, exert pro-angiogenic effects by modulating proliferation and migration of endothelial cells and by stimulating the production of proteases (Lieu et al., 2011; Saylor et al., 2012). Worthy of note, it has been demonstrated that FGF-2 can synergize with both VEGF and PDGF-BB in stimulating neovascularization, this synergism relying on multiple mechanisms. For instance, FGF-2 promotes hypoxia-induced VEGF release by cancer cells and the expression of both VEGF and VEGFRs in endothelial cells, whereas VEGF, in turn, upregulates the expression of FGF-2 (Lieu et al., 2011; Saylor et al., 2012). Moreover, FGF-2 upregulates PDGFRs expression and increases the responsiveness to PDGF-BB in endothelial cells, whereas PDGF-BB enhances FGFR1 expression and FGF-2 responsiveness in vascular smooth muscle cells (Cao et al., 2008; Liu et al., 2011). Remarkably, FGFs are thought to play a critical role in the resistance to anti-VEGF therapy (Lieu et al., 2011; Saylor et al, 2005). Besides, both FGF-1 and -2 may also be involved in tumor cell growth through cell-autonomous, autocrine mechanisms (Kumar-Singh et al., 1999).

FGF-1 and -2 are expressed in the majority of MMs *in vivo* and high levels of FGF-2 in tumor tissues, serum or pleural effusions are associated with a worse prognosis in MM patients (Davidson et al., 2004; Kumar-Singh et al., 1999; Strizzi et al., 2001b). Furthermore, the combined expression levels of FGF-1, FGF-2, VEGF and Transforming Growth Factor beta (TGFβ) in MM tissues correlates with both IMD and a poorer prognosis (Kumar-Singh et al., 1999). In addition to their role in tumor angiogenesis, FGFs act as autocrine growth factors for MM cells. Indeed, MM cells express FGFs and FGF receptors and the transfection with short interfering RNAs to FGF-1 and FGF-2 reduces MM cell proliferation (Kumar-Singh et al., 1999; Liu & Klominek, 2003; Stapelberg et al., 2005). It has also been reported that treatment of MM cells with exogenous FGF-2 stimulates the secretion of matrix metalloproteinases involved in tumor invasion and angiogenesis (Liu & Klominek, 2003).

4. Cross-talk between inflammation and angiogenic growth factors

Experimental and epidemiological evidences indicate that chronic inflammation is associated with most, if not all, tumors and supports their progression (Coussens & Werb 2002; Mantovani et al., 2008; Mantovani et al., 2010; Porta et al., 2009). Chronic inflammation appears to have a versatile function in tumor onset and progression. Indeed, as discussed above, a long-lasting inflammation can contribute to cancer initiation through the production ROS and RNS with DNA-damaging properties. On the other hand, it can also participate in cancer promotion and progression by increasing the availability of mediators (growth factors, cytokines, chemokines, prostaglandins) which contribute to the growth of initiated cells and to neoangiogenesis (Mantovani, 2010). Besides, once a tumor is established, cancer cells promote a constant influx of myelomonocytic cells that express inflammatory mediators supporting pro-tumoral functions. In this regard, myelomonocytic cells are key orchestrators of cancer-related inflammatory processes supporting proliferation and survival of malignant cells, subversion of adaptive immune responses, stromal remodeling and angiogenesis (David Dong et al., 2009; Loges et al., 2009; Porta et al., 2009).

Tissue infiltration by macrophages is a dramatic and common feature of inflammation, angiogenesis and cancer (Pollard, 2004; Sica, 2010). High densities of tumor-infiltrating macrophages are associated with poor survival in patients with MM (Burt et al., 2011). In fact, the recruitment and infiltration of macrophages in the tumor microenvironment can activate them to support the malignant progression of cancer cells. These macrophages are called tumor-associated macrophages (TAMs) (Lawrence, 2011; Sica, 2010). Cancer cells co-cultured with macrophages and incubated with inflammatory cytokines are synergistically stimulated to produce various angiogenesis-related factors (Izzi et al., 2009; Ono, 2008). This inflammatory angiogenesis is mediated, in part, by activation of NF-κB and AP-1 (Angelo & Kurzrock, 2007; Huang et al., 2000; Ono, 2008). In fact, treatment of both vascular endothelial cells and cancer cells with IL-1α/β, TNF-α and ROS *in vitro* results in a marked induction of VEGF and FGF-2, through the transcriptional activation of NF-κB, Specificity protein 1 (Sp-1), AP-1 and hypoxia response elements.

In addition to macrophages, other tumor-infiltrating immune cells including T cells, B cells, natural killer cells and neutrophils can release cytokines, such as IL-1α/β, TNF-α and IL-6, able to sustain the synthesis of angiogenic growth factors (Angelo & Kurzrock, 2007). As for, IL-6, this pro-inflammatory cytokine has been reported to play a critical role in the stimulation of VEGF synthesis by different cell types, including MM cells (Adachi et al., 2006; Angelo & Kurzrock, 2007). Of note, MMs usually produce high levels of IL-6 but express low levels of IL-6R, so that the presence of sIL-6Rs, which may be provided by inflammatory cells recruited to the tumor region, is essential for the IL-6-dependent stimulation of VEGF expression by MM cells (Adachi et al., 2006). Inflammation can also induce the expression of receptors for angiogenic growth factors. In this regard, the expression of PDGFRs is known to be induced by inflammatory cytokines such as TNF-α and IL-1 (Andrae et al., 2008). Besides, inflammatory cells themselves can directly release angiogenic factors such as VEGF, PlGF, FGF-2 and PDGF, among many others, which exert mitogenic and migratory effects on surrounding cells (Sica 2010, Ono 2008). Inflammatory cells recruited in the tumor microenvironment can also produce matrix metalloproteinases which promote the formation of new vessels by degrading the basement membrane and by releasing angiogenic growth factors, such as VEGF, PlGF-2 and FGF-2, stored in the extracellular matrix (Barillari et al.,1998; Cao et al., 2008; Lieu et al., 2011).

The high amount of chemokines/cytokines, growth factors, proteolytic enzymes, proteoglycans, lipid mediators and prostaglandins which is typically found in the tumor microenvironment sustains and exacerbates both inflammation and angiogenesis (Costa et al., 2007; Lin & Karin, 2007; Ono, 2008). In this context, the cross-talk between inflammation and angiogenesis is further corroborated by the evidence that, if on one hand inflammatory mediators have significant effects on angiogenesis, on the other hand angiogenic factors can effectively promote inflammation. As a matter of fact, in addition to their angiogenic role, VEGF and PlGF appear to act as direct proinflammatory mediators in the pathogenesis of different inflammatory conditions (Angelo & Kurzrock, 2007; Yoo et al., 2008). In this regard, VEGF was found to increase the production of TNF-α and IL-6 by human peripheral blood mononuclear cells and macrophages (Yoo et al., 2008). Moreover, VEGF stimulates monocyte recruitment to tumor areas (Barleon et al., 1996). An additional link between inflammatory and angiogenic growth factors has been provided with the demonstration that in myelomonocytic cells TNF-α is upregulated by PlGF in a NFAT1-dependent manner and, in turn, contributes to PlGF-induced myelomonocytic cell recruitment (Ding et al., 2010). PlGF can also contribute to inflammation by acting as survival factor for monocytes and macrophages (Adini et al., 2002).

5. Cooperation between asbestos and angiogenic growth factors in MM onset and progression

As reported above, asbestos stimulates the expression of *c-fos* and *c-jun* mRNA in mesothelial cells in a dose-dependent fashion (Heintz et al., 1993; Ramos-Nino et al., 2002). One of the mechanisms by which VEGF and PlGF elicit biological responses is the induction of Fos-B and c-Fos expression in endothelial cells and monocytes (Holmes & Zachary, 2004). The coexistence of different stimuli, such as asbestos fibers and angiogenic growth factors, concurring to the activation of early response genes might lead to the persistent induction of AP-1 in mesothelial cells and to the chronic stimulation of mesothelial cell proliferation, thus favoring cell transformation.

Further, asbestos and angiogenic growth factors can cooperate in inducing an immunosuppressive tumor microenvironement. Indeed, asbestos has been found to possess immunosuppressive properties. For example, chrysotile fibers have been shown to depress the *in vitro* proliferation of phytohemagglutinin-stimulated peripheral blood lymphocytes and to suppress natural killer activity. Moreover, asbestos significantly reduces the generation and activity of lymphokine-activated killer (LAK) cells, which are immune effectors with a strong lytic activity against MM cells (Manning et al., 1991; Valle et al., 1998).

Immunosuppressive properties have been reported for angiogenic growth factors as well (Ohm et al., 2001; Ziogas et al., 2012). Impaired antigen-presenting function in DCs as a result of abnormal differentiation is an important mechanism of tumor escape from immune control. It has been demonstrated that VEGF can inhibit the maturation of DCs induced by lipopolysaccharide (Takahashi et al., 2004). VEGF can also affect the ability of hematopoetic progenitor cells (HPCs) to differentiate into functional DCs during the early stages of hematopoiesis *in vivo* (Gabrilovich et al., 1996; Oyama et al., 1998). In this regard, it has been shown that VEGF binds to specific receptors on the surface of HPCs and this binding appears to involve VEGF-R1. Interestingly, the number of binding sites available for VEGF decreased with DC maturation and correlated with decreased levels of VEGF-R1 mRNA expression in the late-stage cells (Gabrilovich et al., 1996). PlGF was also found to inhibit the activation and maturation of human DCs effectively and rapidly through the NF-κB pathway (Lin et al., 2007). The results of this study further indicate that by modulating the function of DCs, PlGF can down-regulate T helper immune responses (Lin et al., 2007). In addition, both VEGF and PlGF are also involved in the recruitment of macrophages with immunosuppressive, tumor-promoting roles to the tumor stroma.

On the whole, these findings suggest mechanisms by which tumor-derived soluble factors such as VEGF or PlGF may synergize with asbestos to down-regulate immune responses to MM antigens.

6. Conclusions

Collectively, the reported findings demonstrate that a complex network involving asbestos, inflammation and angiogenic factors upregulation is involved in the pathogenesis of MM. In particular, the abnormal expression of angiogenic factors appears to play multiple roles in MM: it stimulates tumor neovascularization, increases pleural effusion formation by increasing vascular permeability, supports autocrine tumor cell growth and finally, in synergism with asbestos fibers, can sustain inflammation and bias host immune responses. Accordingly, the upregulation of angiogenic growth factors appears to be a crucial event in mesothelial cell transformation and MM progression.

Given the involvement of multiple angiogenic growth growth factors in the formation of tumor vessels, in tumor inflammation and MM cell growth and survival, the therapeutic development of antiangiogenic agents for the treatment of this tumor should be aimed at blocking multiple growth factor signaling pathways and their complex interactive network (Cao et al., 2008; Ikuta et al., 2009; Homsi & Daud, 2007; Lieu et al., 2011).

Author details

Loredana Albonici, Camilla Palumbo and Vittorio Manzari
Department of Experimental Medicine and Biochemical Sciences, University of Rome "Tor Vergata", Rome, Italy

7. References

Adachi, Y., Aoki, C., Yoshio-Hoshino, N., Takayama, K., Curiel, D. T. & Nishimoto N. (2006). Interleukin-6 induces both cell growth and VEGF production in malignant mesotheliomas. *Int. J. Cancer*, Vol. 119, No. 6, (September 2006), pp. 1303-1311, ISSN 0020-7136

Adini, A., Kornaga, T., Firoozbakht, F. & Benjamin, L. E. (2002). Placenta growth factor is a survival factor for human endothelial cells and macrophages. *Cancer Res.*, Vol. 62, No. 10, (May 2002), pp. 2749-2752, ISSN 0008-5472

Albonici, L., Doldo, E., Palumbo, C., Orlandi, A., Bei, R., Pompeo, E., Mineo, T. C., Modesti, A. & Manzari, V. (2009). Placenta growth factor is a survival factor for human malignant mesotelioma cells. *Int. J. Immunopathol. Pharmacol.*, Vol. 22, No. 2, (April-June 2009), pp. 389-401, ISSN 0394-6320

Andrae, J., Gallini, R. & Betsholtz, C. (2008). Role of platelet-derived growth factors in physiology and medicine. *Genes Dev.*, Vol. 22, No. 10, (May 2008), pp. 1276-1312, ISSN 0890-9369

Angelo, L. S. & Kurzrock, R. (2007). Vascular endothelial growth factor and its relationship to inflammatory mediators. *Clin. Cancer Res.*, Vol. 13, No. 10, (May 2007), pp. 2825-2830, ISSN 1078-0432

Antony, V. B., Godbey, S. W., Kunkel, S. L., Hott, J. W., Hartman, D. L., Burdick, M. D. & Strieter, R. M. (1993). Recruitment of inflammatory cells to the pleural space. Chemotactic cytokines, IL-8, and monocyte chemotactic peptide-1 in human pleural fluids. *J. Immunol.*, Vol. 151, No. 12, (December 1993), pp. 7216–7223, ISSN 0022-1767

Asahara, T., Takahashi, T., Masuda, H., Kalka, C., Chen, D., Iwaguro, H., Inai, Y., Silver, M. & Isner, J. M. (1999). VEGF contributes to postnatal neovascularization by mobilizing bone marrow-derived endothelial progenitor cells. *EMBO J.*, Vol. 18, No. 14, (July 1999), pp. 3964-3972, ISSN 0261-4189

Astoul, P. (1999). Pleural mesothelioma. *Curr. Opin. Pulm. Med.*, Vol. 5, No. 4, (July 1999), pp. 259-268, ISSN 1070-5287

Attanoos, R. L. & Gibbs, A. R. (1997). Pathology of malignant mesothelioma. *Histopathology*, Vol. 30, No. 5, (May 1997), pp. 403-418, ISSN 0309-0167

Aust, A. E., Cook, P.M. & Dodson, R. F. (2011). Morphological and chemical mechanisms of elongated mineral particle toxicities. *J. Toxicol. Environ. Health. B Crit. Rev.*, Vol. 14, No. 1-4, pp. 40-75, ISSN 1093-7404

Autiero, M., Waltenberger, J., Communi, D., Kranz, A., Moons, L., Lambrechts, D., Kroll, J., Plaisance, S., De Mol, M., Bono, F., Kliche, S., Fellbrich, G., Ballmer-Hofer, K., Maglione, D., Mayr-Beyrle, U., Dewerchin, M., Dombrowski, S., Stanimirovic, D., Van Hummelen, P., Dehio, C., Hicklin, D. J., Persico, G., Herbert, J. M., Communi, D., Shibuya, M., Collen, D., Conway, E. M. & Carmeliet, P. (2003). Role of PlGF in the intra- and intermolecular cross-talk between the VEGF receptors Flt-1 and Flk-1. *Nat. Med.*, Vol. 9, No. 7, (July 2003), pp. 936-943, ISSN 1078-8956

Baldys, A., Pande, P., Mosleh, T., Park, S. H. & Aust, A. E. (2007). Apoptosis induced by crocidolite asbestos in human lung epithelial cells involves inactivation of Akt and MAPK pathways. *Apoptosis*, Vol. 12, No. 2, (February 2007), pp. 433–447, ISSN 1360-8185

Barillari, G., Albonici, L., Franzese, O., Modesti, A., Liberati, F., Barillari, P., Ensoli, B., Manzari, V. & Santeusanio, G. (1998). The basic residues of placenta growth factor type 2 retrieve sequestered angiogenic factors into soluble form. Implication for tumor angiogenesis. *Am. J. Pathol.*, Vol. 152, No. 5, (May 1998), pp. 1161-1166, ISSN 0002-9440

Barleon, B., Sozzani, S., Zhou, D., Weich, H. A., Mantovani, A. & Marmé, D.(1996). Migration of human monocytes in response to vascular endothelial growth factor (VEGF) is mediated via the VEGF receptor flt-1. *Blood*, Vol. 87, No. 8, (April 1996), pp. 3336-3343, ISSN 0006-4971

Berman, D. W. & Crump, K. S. (2008). A meta-analysis of asbestos-related cancer risk that addresses fiber size and mineral type. *Crit. Rev. Toxicol.*, Vol. 38, Suppl. 1, pp. 49–73, ISSN 1040-8444

BéruBé, K. A., Quinlan, T. R., Fung, H., Magae, J., Vacek, P., Taatjes, D. J. & Mossman, B. T. (1996). Apoptosis is observed in mesothelial cells after exposure to crocidolite asbestos. *Am. J. Respir. Cell. Mol. Biol.*, Vol. 15, No. 1, (July 1996), pp. 141-147, ISSN 1044-1549

Bocchetta, M., Di Resta, I., Powers, A., Fresco, R., Tosolini, A., Testa, J. R., Pass, H.I., Rizzo, P. & Carbone, M. (2000). Human mesothelial cells are unusually susceptible to simian virus 40-mediated transformation and asbestos cocarcinogenicity. *Proc. Natl. Acad. Sci. USA*, Vol. 97, No. 18, (August 2000), pp. 10214–10219, ISSN 0027-8424

Bowie, A. & O'Neill, L. A. (2000). Oxidative stress and nuclear factor-kappaB activation: a reassessment of the evidence in the light of recent discoveries. *Biochem. Pharmacol.*, Vol. 59, No. 1, (January 2000), pp. 13-23, ISSN 0006-2952

Branchaud, R. M., Garant, L. J. & Kane A. B. (1993). Pathogenesis of mesothelial reactions to asbestos fibers. Monocyte recruitment and macrophage activation. *Pathobiology*, Vol. 61, No. 3-4, pp. 154–163, ISSN 1015-2008

Broaddus, V. C., Yang, L., Scavo, L. M., Ernst, J. D. & Boylan, A. M. (1996). Asbestos induces apoptosis of human and rabbit pleural mesothelial cells via reactive oxygen species. *J. Clin. Invest.*, Vol. 98, No. 9, (November 1996), pp. 2050–2059, ISSN 0021-9738

Brown, D., Beswick, P. & Donaldson, K. (1999). Induction of nuclear translocation of NF-κB in epithelial cells by respirable mineral fibres. *J. Pathol.*, Vol. 189, No. 2, (October 1999), pp. 258–264, ISSN 0022-3417

Burt, B. M., Rodig, S. J., tilleman, T. R., Elbardissi, A. W., Bueno, R., Sugarbaker, D. J. (2011). Circulating and tumor-infiltrating myeloid cells predict survival in human pleural mesothelioma. *Cancer*, Vol. 117, No. 22, (November 2011), pp. 5234-5244, ISSN 0008-543X

Cacciotti, P., Strizzi, L., Vianale, G., Iaccheri, L., Libener, R., Porta, C., Tognon, M., Gaudino, G. & Mutti, L. (2002). The presence of simian-virus 40 sequences in mesothelioma and mesothelial cells is associated with high levels of vascular growth factor. *Am. J. Respir. Cell. Mol. Biol.*, Vol. 26, No. 2, (February 2002), pp. 189-193, ISSN 1044-1549

Cao, Y., Cao, R. & Hedlund, E. M. (2008). R Regulation of tumor angiogenesis and metastasis by FGF and PDGF signaling pathways. *J Mol. Med. (Berl.)*, Vol. 86, No. 7, (July 2008), pp. 785-789, ISSN 0946-2716

Cao, Y., Chen, H., Zhou, L., Chiang, M. K., Anand-Apte, B., Weatherbee, J. A., Wang, Y., Fang, F., Flanagan, J. G. & Tsang, M. L. (1996). Heterodimers of placenta growth factor/vascular endothelial growth factor. Endothelial activity, tumor cell expression, and high affinity binding to Flk-1/KDR. *J. Biol. Chem.*, Vol. 271, No. 6, (February 1996), pp. 3154-3162, ISSN 0021-9258

Carbone, M., Kratzke, R. A. & Testa, J. R. (2002). The pathogenesis of mesothelioma. *Semin. Oncol.*, Vol. 29, No. 1, (February 2002), pp. 2-17, ISSN 0093-7754

Carbone, M., Ly, B. H., Dodson, R. F., Pagano, I., Morris, P. T., Dogan, U. A., Gazdar, A. F., Pass, H. I. & Yang, H. (2012). Malignant mesothelioma: Facts, myths and hypotheses. *J. Cell. Physiol.*, Vol. 227, No. 1 (January 2012), pp. 44-58, ISSN 0021-9541

Carmeliet, P. (2003). Angiogenesis in health and disease. *Nat. Med.*, Vol. 9, No. 6, (June 2003), pp. 653-660, ISSN 1078-8956

Carmeliet. P., Moons, L., Luttun, A., Vincenti, V., Compernolle, V., De Mol, M., Wu, Y., Bono, F., Devy, L., Beck, H., Scholz, D., Acker, T., DiPalma, T., Dewerchin, M., Noel, A., Stalmans, I., Barra, A., Blacher, S., Vandendriessche, T., Ponten, A., Eriksson, U., Plate, K. H., Foidart, J. M., Schaper, W., Charnock-Jones, D. S., Hicklin, D. J., Herbert, J. M., Collen, D. & Persico, M. G. (2001). Synergism between vascular endothelial growth factor and placental growth factor contributes to angiogenesis and plasma extravasation in pathological conditions. *Nat. Med.*, Vol. 7, No. 5, (May 2001), pp. 575-583, ISSN 1078-8956

Catalano, A., Lazzarini, R., Di Nuzzo, S., Orciari, S. & Procopio A. (2009). The plexin-A1 receptor activates vascular endothelial growth factor-receptor 2 and nuclear factor-kappaB to mediate survival and anchorage-independent growth of malignant mesothelioma cells. *Cancer Res.*, Vol. 69, No. 4, (February 2009), pp. 1485-1493, ISSN 0008-5472

Catalano, A., Romano, M., Martinotti, S. & Procopio, A. (2002). Enhanced expression of vascular endothelial growth factor (VEGF) plays a critical role in the tumor progression potential induced by simian virus 40 large T antigen. *Oncogene*, Vol. 21, No. 18 (April 2002), pp. 2896-2900, ISSN 0950-9232

Chang, L. & Karin, M. (2001). Mammalian MAP kinase signalling cascades. *Nature*, Vol. 410, No. 6824, (March 2001), pp. 37–40, ISSN 0028-0836

Chen, C. N., Hsieh, F. J., Cheng, Y. M., Cheng, W. F., Su, Y. N., Chang, K. J. & Lee, P. H. (2004). The significance of placenta growth factor in angiogenesis and clinical outcome of human gastric cancer. *Cancer Lett.*, Vol. 213, No. 1, (September 2004), pp. 73-82, ISSN 0304-3835

Cheng, N., Shi, X., Ye, J., Castranova, V., Chen, F., Leonard, S. S., Vallyathan, V. & Rojanasakul, Y. (1999). Role of transcription factor NF-kappaB in asbestos-induced TNFalpha response from macrophages. *Exp. Mol. Pathol.*, Vol. 66, No. 3, (August 1999), pp. 201-210, ISSN 0014-4800

Choe, N., Tanaka, S., Xia, W., Hemenway, D. R., Roggli, V. L. & Kagan, E. (1997). Pleural macrophage recruitment and activation in asbestos-induced pleural injury. *Environ. Health Perspect.*, Vol. 105, Suppl. 5, (September 1997), pp. 1257-1260, ISSN 0091-6765

Choi, C. H., Song, S. Y., Choi, J. J., Park, Y. A., Kang, H., Kim, T. J., Lee, J. W., Kim, B. G., Lee, J. H. & Bae, D. S. (2008). Prognostic significance of VEGF expression in patients with bulky cervical carcinoma undergoing neoadjuvant chemotherapy. *BMC Cancer*, Vol. 8, (October 2008), p. 295, ISSN 1471-2407

Costa, C., Incio, J. & Soares, R. (2007). Angiogenesis and chronic inflammation: cause or consequence? *Angiogenesis*, Vol. 10, No. 3, pp. 149–166, ISSN 0969-6970

Coussens, L. M. & Werb, Z. (2002). Inflammation and cancer. *Nature*, Vol. 420, No. 6917, (December 2002), pp. 860–867, ISSN 0028-0836

David Dong, Z. M., Aplin, A. C. & Nicosia, R. F. (2009). Regulation of angiogenesis by macrophages, dendritic cells, and circulating myelomonocytic cells. *Curr. Pharm. Des.*, Vol. 15, No. 4, pp. 365-379, ISSN 1381-6128

Davidson, B., Vintman, L., Zcharia, E., Bedrossian, C., Berner, A., Nielsen, S., Ilan, N., Vlodavsky, I & Reich, R. (2004). Heparanase and basic fibroblast growth factor are co-expressed in malignant mesothelioma. *Clin. Exp. Metastasis*, Vol. 21, No. 5, pp. 469-476, ISSN 0262-0898

Dawson, M. R., Duda, D. G., Fukumura, D. & Jain, R. K. (2009). VEGFR1-activity-independent metastasis formation. *Nature*, Vol. 461, No. 7262, (September 2009), pp. E4-E5, ISSN 0028-0836.

Ding, Y., Huang, Y., Song, N. Gao, X., Yuan, S., Wang, X., Cai, H., Fu, Y. & Luo, Y. (2010). NFAT1 mediates placental growth factor-induced myelomonocytic cell recruitment via the induction of TNF-alpha. *J. Immunol.*, Vol. 184, No. 5, (March 2010), pp. 2593-2601, ISSN 0022-1767

Dong, H. Y., Buard, A., Renier, A., Levy, F., Saint-Etienne, L. & Jaurand, M. C. (1994). Role of oxygen derivatives in the cytotoxicity and DNA damage produced by asbestos on rat pleural mesothelial cells in vitro. *Carcinogenesis,* Vol. 15, No. 6, (June 1994), pp. 1251–1255, ISSN 0143-3334

Dorai, T., Kobayashi, H.; Holland, J. F. & Onhuma, T. (1994). Modulation of platelet-derived growth factor-beta mRNA expression and cell growth in a human mesothelioma cell line by a hammerhead ribozyme. *Mol. Pharmacol.*, Vol. 46, No. 3, (September 1994, pp. 437-444, ISSN 0026-895X

Driscoll, K., Carter, J., Howard, B., Hassenbein, D., Janssen, Y. & Mossman, B. T. (1998). Crocidolite activates NF-κB and MIP-2 gene expression in rat alveolar epithelial cells. Role of mitochondrial-derived oxidants. *Environ. Health Perspect.,* Vol. 106, Suppl. 5, (October 1998), pp. 1171–1174, ISSN 0091-6765

Eferl, R., & Wagner, E. F.(2003). AP1: a double-edged sword in tumorigenesis. *Nature Rev. Cancer,* Vol. 3, No. 11, (November 2003), pp. 859–868, ISSN 1474-175X

Fennell, D. A. & Rudd, R. M. (2004). Defective core-apoptosis signaling in diffuse malignant pleural mesothelioma: opportunities for effective drug development. *Lancet Oncol.*, Vol. 5, No. 6, (June 2004), pp. 354-362, ISSN 1470-2045

Ferrara, N., Gerber, H. P. & LeCouter, J. (2003). The biology of VEGF and its receptors. *Nat. Med.*, Vol. 9, No. 6, (June 2003), pp. 669-676, ISSN 1078-8956

Filiberti, R., Marroni, P., Neri, M., Ardizzoni, A., Betta P. G., Cafferata, M. A., Canessa, P. A., Puntoni, R., Ivaldi, G. P., & Paganuzzi, M. (2005). Serum PDGF-AB in pleural mesotelioma. *Tumour Biol.*, Vol. 26, No. 5, (September-October 2005), pp. 221-226, ISSN 1010-4283

Fischer, C., Jonckx, B., Mazzone, M., Zacchigna, S., Loges, S., Pattarini, L., Chorianopoulos, E., Liesenborghs, L., Kock M., De Mol, M., Autiero, M., Wyns, S., Plaisance, S., Moons, L., van Rooijen, N., Giacca, M., Stassen J. M., Dewerchin, M., Collen, D. & Carmeliet, P. (2007). Anti-PlGF inhibits growth of VEGF(R)-inhibitor-resistant tumors without affecting healthy vessels. *Cell*, Vol. 131, No. 3, (November 2007), pp. 463-475, ISSN 0092-8674

Fischer, C., Mazzone, M., Jonckx, B. & Carmeliet, P. (2008). FLT1 and its ligands VEGFB and PlGF: drug targets for anti-angiogenic therapy? *Nat. Rev. Cancer.*, Vol. 8, No. 12, (December 2008), pp. 942-956, ISSN 1474-175X

Fleury-Feith, J., Pilatte, Y. & Jaurand, M. C. (2003). Cells in the pleural cavity, In: *Textbook of pleural diseases*, Light, R. W. & Lee, Y. C. G., pp. 17-34, Arnold Publishers, ISBN 9780340807941, London.

Folkman, J. (2006). Angiogenesis. *Annu. Rev. Med.*, Vol. 57, pp. 1–18, ISSN 0066-4219

Gabrilovich, D. I., Chen, H. L., Girgis, K. R., Cunningham, H. T., Meny, G. M., Nadaf, S., Kavanaugh, D. & Carbone, D. P. (1996). Production of vascular endothelial growth factor by human tumors inhibits the functional maturation of dendritic cells. *Nat. Med.*, Vol. 2, No. 10, (October 1996), pp. 1096-1103, ISSN 1078-8956

Garlepp, M. J & Leong, C. C. (1995). Biological and immunological aspects of malignant mesothelioma. *Eur. Respir. J.*, Vol. 8, No. 4, (April 1995), pp. 643-650, ISSN 0903-1936

Gasparini, G. & Harris, A. L. (1995). Clinical importance of the determination of tumor angiogenesis in breast carcinoma: much more than a new prognostic tool. *J. Clin. Oncol.*, Vol. 13, No. 3, (March 1995), pp. 765-782, ISSN 0732-183X

Gazdar, A. F. & Carbone, M. (2003). Molecular pathogenesis of malignant mesothelioma and its relationship to simian virus 40. *Clin. Lung Cancer*, Vol. 5, No. 3, (November 2003), pp. 177-181, ISSN 1525-7304

Gossart, S., Cambon, C., Orfila , C., Séquélas, M. H., Lepert, J. C., Rami, J., Carrè, P. & Pipy, B. (1996). Reactive oxygen intermediated as regulators of TNF-alpha production in rat lung inflammation induced by silica. *J. Immunol.*, Vol. 156, No. 4, (February 1996), pp. 1540-1548, ISSN 0022-1767

Greillier, L. & Astoul, P. (2008). Mesothelioma and asbestos-related pleural diseases. *Respiration*, Vol. 76, No. 1, pp. 1-15, ISSN 0025-7931

Gulumian, M. (2005). An update on the detoxification processes for silica particles and asbestos fibers: successess and limitations. *J. Toxicol. Environ. Health. B Crit. Rev.*, Vol. 8, No. 6, (November-December 2005), pp. 453-483, ISSN 1093-7404

Haegens, A., Barrett, T. F., Gell, J., Shukla, A., Macpherson, M., Vacek, P., Poynter, M. E., Butnor, K. J., Janssen-Heininger, Y. M., Steele, C. & Mossman, B. T. (2007). Airway epithelial NF-kappaB activation modulates asbestos-induced inflammation and mucin production in vivo. *J. Immunol.*, Vol. 178, No. 3, (February 2007), pp. 1800-1808, ISSN 0022-1767

Harmey, J. H. & Bouchier-Hayes, D. (2002). Vascular endothelial growth factor (VEGF), a survival factor for tumour cells: implications for anti-angiogenic therapy. *Bioessays*, Vol. 24, No. 3, (March 2002), pp. 280-283, ISSN 0265-9247

Hattori, K., Heissig, B., Wu, Y., Dias, S., Tejada, R., Ferris, B., Hicklin, D. J., Zhu, Z., Bohlen, P., Witte, L., Hendrikx, J., Hackett, N. R., Crystal, R. G., Moore, M. A., Werb, Z., Lyden, D. & Rafii, S. (2002). Placental growth factor reconstitutes hematopoiesis by recruiting VEGFR1(+) stem cells from bone-marrow microenvironment. *Nat. Med.*, Vol. 8, No. 8, (August 2002), pp. 841-849, ISSN 1078-8956

Hausmann, M. J., Rogachev, B., Weiler, M., Chaimovitz, C. & Douvdevani, A. (2000). Accessory role of human peritoneal mesothelial cells in antigen presentation and T-cell growth. *Kidney Int.*, Vol. 57, No. 2, (February 2000), pp. 476–86, ISSN 0085-2538

Hayden, M. S. & Gosh, S. (2004). Signaling to NF-κB. *Genes Dev.*, Vol. 18, No. 18, (Spetember 2004), pp. 2195-2224, ISSN 0890-9369

Hayden, M. S. & Ghosh, S. (2008). Shared principles in NF-kappaB signaling. *Cell*, Vol. 132, No. 3, (February 2008), pp. 344–362, ISSN 0092-8674

Heintz, N. H., Janssen, Y. M. & Mossman, B. T. (1993). Persistent induction of c-fos and c-jun expression by asbestos. *Proc. Natl. Acad. Sci. USA*, Vol. 90, No. 8, (April 1993), pp. 3299–3303, ISSN 0027-8424

Heintz, N. H., Janssen-Heininger, Y. M. & Mossman, B. T. (2010). Asbestos, lung cancers, and mesotheliomas: from molecular approaches to targeting tumor survival pathways. *Am. J. Respir. Cell Mol. Biol.*, Vol. 42, No. 2, (February 2010), pp. 133–139, ISSN 1044-1549

Hillegass, J. M., Shukla, A., Lathrop, S. A., MacPherson, M. B., Beuschel, S. L., Butnor, K. J., Testa, J. R., Pass, H. I., Carbone, M., Steele, C. & Mossman, B. T. (2010). Inflammation precedes the development of human malignant mesotheliomas in a SCID mouse xenograft model. *Ann. N. Y. Acad. Sci.*, Vol. 1203, (August 2010), pp. 7-14, ISSN 0077-8923

Hirayama, N., Tabata, C., Tabata, R., Maeda, R., Yasumitsu, A., Yamada, S., Kuribayashi, K., Fukuoka, K. & Nakano T. (2011). Pleural effusion VEGF levels as a prognostic factor of malignant pleural mesothelioma. *Respir. Med.*, Vol. 105, No. 1 (January 2011), pp. 137-142, ISSN 0954-6111

Hoffmann, A., Natoli, G. & Baltimore, D. (2003). Genetic analysis of NF-kappaB/Rel transcription factor defines functional specificities. *EMBO J.*, Vol. 22, No. 20, (October 2003), pp. 5530-5539, ISSN 0261-4189

Hoffmann, A., Natoli, G. & Ghosh, G. (2006). Transcriptional regulation via the NF-kappaB signaling module. Oncogene, Vol. 25, No. 51, (October 2006), pp. 6706-6716, ISSN 0950-9232

Hoidal, J. R. (2001). Reactive oxygen species and cell signaling. *Am. J. Respir. Cell Mol. Biol.*, Vol. 25, No. 6, (December 2001), pp. 661–663, ISSN 1044-1549

Holmes, D. I. & Zachary, I. (2004). Placental growth factor induces FosB and c-Fos gene expression via Flt-1 receptors. *FEBS Lett.*, Vol. 557, No. 1-3, (January 2004), pp. 93-98, ISSN 0014-5793

Homsi, J. & Daud, A. I. (2007). Spectrum of activity and mechanism of action of VEGF/PDGF inhibitors. *Cancer Control*, vol. 14, No. 3, (July 2007), pp. 285-294, ISSN 1073-2748

Huang, S., Robinson, J. B., Deguzman, A., Bucana, C. D. & Fidler, I. J. (2000). Blockade of nuclear factor-kappaB signaling inhibits angiogenesis and tumorigenicity of human ovarian cancer cells by suppressing expression of vascular endothelial growth factor and interleukin 8. *Cancer Res.*, Vol. 60, No. 19, (October 2000), pp. 5334–5539, ISSN 0008-5472

Huang, S. X., Jaurand, M. C., Kamp, D. W., Whysner, J. & Hei, T. K. (2011). Role of mutagenicity in asbestos fiber-induced carcinogenicity and other diseases. *J. Toxicol. Environ. Health B. Crit. Rev.*, Vol. 14, No. 1-4, pp. 179-245, ISSN 1093-7404

Hussain, S. P., Hofseth, L. J. & Harris, C. C. (2003). Radical causes of cancer. *Nat. Rev. Cancer.*, Vol. 3, No. 4, (April 2003), pp. 276-285, ISSN 1474-175X

Ikuta, K., Yano, S., Trung, V. T., Hanibuchi, M., Goto, H., Li, Q., Wang, W., Yamada, T., Ogino, H., Kakiuchi, S., Uehara, H., Sekido, Y., Uenaka, T., Nishioka, Y & Sone, S. (2009). E7080, a multi-tyrosine kinase inhibitor, suppresses the progression of malignant pleural mesothelioma with different proangiogenic cytokine production profiles. *Clin. Cancer Res.*, Vol. 15, No. 23, (December 2009), pp. 7229-7237, ISSN 1078-0432

Izzi, V., Chiurchiù, V., D'Aquilio, F., Palumbo, C., Tresoldi, I., Modesti, A. & Baldini, P. M. (2009). Differential effects of malignant mesothelioma cells on THP-1 monocytes and macrophages. *Int. J. Oncol.*, Vol. 34, No. 2, (February 2009), pp. 543-550, ISSN 1019-6439

Janssen-Heininger, Y. M., Macara, I. & Mossman, B. T. (1999). Cooperativity between oxidants and tumor necrosis factor in the activation of nuclear factor (NF)-kappaB: requirement of Ras/mitogen-activated protein kinases in the activation of NF-kappaB by oxidants. *Am. J. Respir. Cell. Mol. Biol.*, Vol. 20, No. 5, (May 1999), pp. 942-952, ISSN 1044-1549

Janssen, Y. M., Barchowsky, A., Treadwell, M., Driscoll, K. E. & Mossman, B. T. (1995). Asbestos induces nuclear factor-κB (NF-κB) DNA-binding activity and NF-κB-dependent gene expression in tracheal epithelial cells. *Proc. Natl. Acad. Sci. USA*, Vol. 92, No. 18, (August 1995), pp. 8458–8462, ISSN 0027-8424

Janssen, Y. M., Driscoll, K. E., Howard, B., Quinlan, T. R., Treadwell, M., Barchowsky, A. & Mossman, B. T. (1997). Asbestos causes translocation of p65 protein and increases NF-kappa B DNA binding activity in rat lung epithelial and pleural mesothelial cells. *Am. J. Pathol.*, Vol. 151, No. 2, (August 1997), pp. 389–401, ISSN 0002-9440

Jash, A., Sahoo, A., Kim, G. C., Chae, C. S., Hwang, J. S., Kim, J. E. & Im, S. H. (2012). Nuclear factor of activated T cells 1 (NFAT1) induced permissive chromatin modification facilitates nuclear Factor-κB (NF-κB) mediated interleukin-9 (IL-9) transactivation. *J. Biol. Chem.*, (March 2012), Epub ahead of print, ISSN 1083-351X

Jochum, W., Passegué, E. & Wagner, E. F. (2001). AP-1 in mouse development and tumorigenesis. *Oncogene*, Vol. 20, No. 19, (April 2001), pp. 2401-2412, ISSN 0950-9232

Jung, Y. J., Isaacs, J. S., Lee, S., Trepel, J. & Neckers, L. (2003). IL-1beta-mediated up-regulation of HIF-1alpha via an NF-kappaB/COX-2 pathway identifies HIF-1 as a critical link between inflammation and oncogenesis. *FASEB J.*, Vol. 17, No. 14, (November 2003), pp. 2115-2117, ISSN 0892-6638

Kamp, D. W. & Weitzman, S. A. (1999). The molecular basis of asbestos induced lung injury. *Thorax*, Vol. 54, No. 7, (July 1999), pp. 638-652, ISSN 0040-6376

Kanwar, J. R., Kamalapuram, S. K. & Kanwar, R. K. (2011). Targeting surviving in cancer: the cell-signalling perspective. *Drug Discov. Today*, Vol. 16, No. 11-12, (June 2011), pp. 485-494, ISSN 1359-6446

Kerbel, R. S. (2008). Tumor angiogenesis. *N. Engl. J. Med.*, Vol. 358, No. 19, (May 2008), pp. 2039-2049, ISSN 0028-4793

Kerber, M., Reiss, Y., Wickersheim, A., Jugold, M., Kiessling, F., Heil, M., Tchaikovski, V., Waltenberger, J., Shibuya, M., Plate, K. H. & Machein, M. R. (2008).Flt-1 signaling in macrophages promotes glioma growth in vivo. *Cancer Res.*, Vol. 68, No. 18, (September 2008), pp. 7342-7351, ISSN 0008-5472

Khaliq, A., Li, X. F., Shams, M., Sisi, P., Acevedo, C. A., Whittle, M. J., Weich, H. & Ahmed, A. (1996). Localization of placenta growth factor (PlGF) in human term placenta. *Growth Factors*, Vol. 13, No. 3-4, pp. 243-250, ISSN 0897-7194

Knights, V. & Cook, S. J. (2010). De-regulated FGF receptors as therapeutic targets in cancer. *Pharmacol. Ther.*, Vol. 125, No. 1, (January 2010), pp. 105-117, ISSN 0163-7258

Koch, S., Tugues, S., Li, X., Gualandi, L. & Claesson-Welsh, L. (2011). Signal transduction by vascular endothelial growth factor receptors. *Biochem J.*, Vol. 437, No. 2, (July 2011), pp. 169-183, ISSN 0264, 6021

Kothmaier, H., Quehenberger, F., Halbewedl, I., Morbini, P., Demirag, F., Zeren, H., Comin, C. E., Murer, B., Cagle, P. T., Attanoos, R., Gibbs, A. R., Galateau-Salle, F. & Popper, H. H. (2008). EGFR and PDGFR differentially promote growth in malignant epithelioid mesothelioma of short and long term survivors. *Thorax*, Vol. 63, No. 4, (April 2008), pp. 345-351, ISSN 0040-6376

Kumar, S., Guleria, R., Singh, V., Bharti, A. C., Mohan, A. & Das, B. C. (2009). Efficacy of plasma vascular endothelial growth factor in monitoring first-line chemotherapy in patients with advanced non-small cell lung cancer. *BMC Cancer*, Vol. 9, (December 2009), p. 421, ISSN 1471-2407

Kumar-Singh, S., Vermuelen, P. B., Weyler, J., Segers, K., Wejn, B., Van Daele, A., Dirix, L. Y., Van Oosterom, A. T. & Van Mark, E. (1997). Evalutation of tumor angiogenesis as a prognostic marker in malignant mesothelioma. *J. Pathol.*, Vol. 182, No. 2, (June 1997), pp. 211-216, ISSN 0022-3417

Kumar-Singh, S., Weyler, J., Martin, M. J., Vermeulen, P. B. & Van Marck, E. (1999). Angiogenic cytokines in mesothelioma: a study of VEGF, FGF-1 and -2, and TGF beta expression. *J. Pathol.*, Vol. 189, No. 1, (September 1999), pp. 72-82, ISSN 0022-3417

Langerak, A. W., van der Linden-van Beurden, C. A. & Versnel, M. A. (1996a). Regulation of differential expression of platelet-derived growth factor alpha- and beta-receptor mRNA in normal and malignant human mesothelial cell lines. *Biochim. Biophys. Acta.*, Vol. 1305, No. 1-2, (February 1996), pp. 63-70, ISSN 0006-3002

Langerak, A. W., De Laat, P. A., Van Der Linden-Van Beurden, C. A., Delahaye, M., Van Der Kwast, T. H., Hoogsteden, H. C., Benner, R. & Versnel, M. A. (1996b). Expression of platelet-derived growth factor (PDGF) and PDGF receptors in human malignant mesothelioma in vitro and in vivo. *J. Pathol.*, Vol. 178, No. 2, (February 1996), pp. 151-160, ISSN 0022-3417

Lawrence, T. (2011). Macrophages and NF-κB in cancer. *Curr. Top. Microbiol. Immunol.*, Vol. 349, pp. 171-184, ISSN 0070-217X

Lemaire, I. & Ouellet, S. (1996). Distinctive profile of alveolar macrophage-derived cytokine release induced by fibrogenic and nonfibrogenic mineral dusts. *J. Toxicol. Environ. Health.*, Vol. 47, No. 5, (April 1996), pp. 465-478, ISSN 0098-4108

Le Page, C., Koumakpayi, I. H., Lessard, L., Mes-Masson, A. M. & Saad, F. (2005). EGFR and Her-2 regulate the constitutive activation of NF-kappaB in PC-3 prostate cancer cells. *Prostate*, Vol. 65, No. 2, (October 2005), pp. 130-140, ISSN 0270-4137

Li, J., Huang, B., Shi, X., Castranova, V., Vallyathan, V. & Huang, C. (2002). Involvement of hydrogen peroxide in asbestos-induced NFAT activation. *Mol. Cell. Biochem.*, Vol. 234–235, No. 1-2, (May-June 2002), pp. 161–168, ISSN 0300-8177

Li, Q., Wang,, W., Yamada, T., Matsumoto, K., Sakai, K., Bando, Y., Uehara, H., Nishioka, Y., Sone, S., Iwakiri, S., Itoi, K., Utsugi, T., Yasumoto, K. & Yano, S. (2011). Pleural mesothelioma instigates tumor-associated fibroblasts to promote progression via a malignant cytokine network. *Am. J. Pathol.*, Vol. 179, No. 3, (September 2011), pp. 1483-1493, ISSN 0002-9440

Lieu, C., Heymach, J., Overman, M., Tran, H. & Kopetz, S. (2011). Beyond VEGF: inhibition of the fibroblast growth factor pathway and antiangiogenesis. *Clin. Cancer Res.*, Vol. 17, No. 19, (October 2011), pp. 6130-6139, ISSN 1078-0432

Lin, Y. L., Liang, Y. C. & Chiang, B. L. (2007). Placental growth factor down-regulates type 1 T helper immune response by modulating the function of dendritic cells. *J. Leukoc. Biol.*, Vol. 82, No. 6, (December 2007), pp. 1473-1480, ISSN 0741-5400

Lin, W. W. & Karin, M. (2007). A cytokine-mediated link between inmate immunity, inflammation, and cancer. *J. Clin. Invest.*, Vol. 117, No. 5, (May 2007), pp. 1175–1182, ISSN 0021-9738

Liu, W., Ernst, J. D. & Broaddus, V. C. (2000). Phagocytosis of crocidolite asbestos induces oxidative stress, DNA damage, and apoptosis in mesothelial cells. *Am. J. Respir. Cell. Mol. Biol.*, vol. 23, No. 3, (September 2000), pp. 371-378, ISSN 1044-1549

Liu, Z. & Klominek, J. (2003). Regulation of matrix metalloprotease activity in malignant mesothelioma cell lines by growth factors. *Thorax*, Vol. 58, No. 3, (March 2003), pp. 198-203, ISSN 0040-6376

Loges, S., Schmidt, T, & Carmeliet, P. (2009). "Antimyeloangiogenic" therapy for cancer by inhibiting PlGF. *Clin. Cancer Res.*, Vol. 15, No. 11, (June 2009), pp. 3648-3653, ISSN 1078-0432

Luttun, A., Tjwa, M. & Carmeliet, P. (2002). Placenta growth factor (PlGF) and its receptor Flt-1 (VEGFR-1): novel therapeutic targets for angiogenic disorders. *Ann. N. Y. Acad. Sci.*, Vol. 979, (December 2002), pp. 80-93, ISSN 0077-8923

Macian, F. (2005). NFAT proteins: key regulators of T-cell development and function. *Nature Rev. Immunol.*, Vol. 5, No. 6, (June 2005), pp. 472–484, ISSN 1474-1733.

Macián, F., López-Rodríguez, C., & Rao. A. (2001). Partners in transcription: NFAT and AP-1. *Oncogene*, Vol. 20, No. 19, (April 2001), pp. 2476-2489, ISSN 0950-9232

Maglione, D., Guerriero, V., Viglietto, G., Delli-Bovi, P. & Persico, M. G. (1991). Isolation of a human placenta cDNA coding for a protein related to the vascular permeability factor. *Proc. Natl. Acad. Sci. USA*, Vol. 88, No. 20, (October 1991), pp. 9267-9271, ISSN 0027-8424

Mancini, M. & Toker, A. (2009). NFAT proteins: emerging roles in cancer progression. *Nature Rev. Cancer.*, Vol. 9, No. 11, (November 2009), pp. 810–820, ISSN 1474-175X

Manning, C. B., Vallyathan, V. & Mossman, B. T. (2002). Diseases caused by asbestos: mechanisms of injury and disease development. *Int. Immunopharmacol.*, Vol. 2, No. 2-3, (February 2002), pp. 191-200, ISSN 1567-5769

Manning, L. S., Davis, M. R. & Robinson, B. W. (1991). Asbestos fibres inhibit the in vitro activity of lymphokine-activated killer (LAK) cells from healthy individuals and patients with malignant mesothelioma. *Clin. Exp. Immunol.*, Vol. 83, No. 1, (January 1991), pp. 85-91, ISSN 0009-9104

Mantovani, A. (2010). Molecular pathways linking inflammation and cancer. *Curr. Mol. Med.*, Vol. 10, No. 4, (June 2010), pp. 369-373, ISSN 1566-5240

Mantovani, A., Allavena, P., Sica, A., & Balkwill, F. (2008). Cancer-related inflammation. *Nature*, Vol. 454, No. 7203, (July 2008), pp. 436-444, ISSN 0028-0836

Marcellini, M., De Luca, N., Riccioni, T., Ciucci, A., Orecchia, A., Lacal, P. M., Ruffini, F., Pesce, M., Cianfarani, F., Zambruno, G., Orlandi, A. & Failla, M. C. (2006). Increased melanoma growth and metastasis spreading in mice overexpressing placenta growth factor. *Am. J. Pathol.,* Vol. 169, No. 2, (August 2006), pp. 643-654, ISSN 0002-9440

Masood, R., Cai, J., Zheng, T., Smith, D. L., Hinton, D. R. & Gill, P. S. (2001). Vascular endothelial growth factor (VEGF) is an autocrine growth factor for VEGF receptor-positive human tumors. *Blood,* Vol. 98, No. 6, (September 2001), pp. 1904-1913, ISSN 0006-4971

Metheny-Barlow, L. J., Flynn, B., van Gijssel, H.E., Marrogi, A. & Gerwin, B. I. (2001). Paradoxical effects of platelet-derived growth factor-A overexpression in malignant mesothelioma. Antiproliferative effects in vitro and tumorigenic stimulation in vivo. *Am. J. Respir. Cell Mol. Biol.*, Vol. 24, No. 6, (June 2001), pp. 694-702, ISSN 1044-1549

Micheau, O. & Tschopp, J. (2003). Induction of TNF receptor I-mediated apoptosis via two sequential signaling complexes. *Cell,* Vol. 114, No. 2, (July 2003), pp. 181-190, ISSN 0092-8674

Milde-Langosch, K. (2005). The Fos family of transcription factors and their role in tumourigenesis. *Eur. J. Cancer.*, Vol. 41, No. 16, (November 2005), pp. 2449-2461, ISSN 0014-2964

Miura, Y., Nishimura, Y., Katsuyama, H., Maeda, M., Hayashi, H., Dong, M., Hyodoh, F., Tomita, M., Matsuo, Y., Uesaka, A., Kuribayashi, K., Nakano, T., Kishimoto, T. & Otsuki T. (2006). Involvement of IL-10 and Bcl-2 in resistance against an asbestos-induced apoptosis of T cells. *Apoptosis,* Vol. 11, No. 10, (October 2006), pp. 1825–1835, ISSN 1360-8185

Mossman, B. T. & Churg, A. (1998). Mechanisms in the pathogenesis of asbestosis and silicosis. *Am. J. Respir. Crit. Care Med.,* Vol. 157, No. 5, (May 1998), pp. 1666-1680, ISSN 1073-449X

Müller, M. R. & Rao, A. (2010). NFAT, immunity and cancer: a transcription factor comes of age. *Nat. Rev. Immunol.,* Vol. 10, No. 9, (September 2010), pp. 645-656, ISSN 1474-1733

Mutsaers, S,E. (2002). Mesothelial cells: Their structure, function and role in serosal repair. *Respirology,* Vol. 7, No. 3, (September 2002), pp. 171–191, ISSN 1323-7799

Mutsaers, S. E. (2004). The mesothelial cell. *Int. J. Biochem. Cell Biol.,* Vol. 36, No. 1, (January 2004), pp. 9-16, ISSN 1357-2725

Nymark, P., Lindholm, P. M., Korpela, M. V., Lahti, L., Ruosaari, S., Kaski, S., Hollmén. J., Anttila, S., Kinnula, V. L. & Knuutila, S. (2007). Gene expression profiles in asbestos-exposed epithelial and mesothelial lung cell lines. *BMC Genomics,* Vol. 8, (March 2007), p. 62, ISSN 1471-2164

Ohm, J. E. & Carbone, D. P. (2001). VEGF as a mediator of tumor-associated immunodeficiency. *Immunol. Res.*, Vol. 23, No. 2-3, pp. 263-272, ISSN 0257-277X

Ohta, Y., Shridhar, V., Bright, R. K., Kalemkerian, G. P., Du, W., Carbone, M., Watanabe, Y. & Pass, H. I. (1999). VEGF and VEGF type C play an important role in angiogenesis and lymphangiogenesis in human malignant mesothelioma tumours. *Br. J. Cancer.*, Vol. 81, No. 1, (September 1999), pp. 54–61, ISSN 0007-0920

Olsson, A. K., Dimberg, A., Kreuger, J. & Claesson-Welsh, L. (2006). VEGF receptor signaling – in control of vascular function. *Nat. Rev. Mol. Cell. Biol.*, Vol. 7, No. 5, (May 2006), pp. 359-371, ISSN 1471-0072

Ono, M. (2008). Molecular links between tumor angiogenesis and inflammation: inflammatory stimuli of macrophages and cancer cells as targets for therapeutic strategy. *Cancer Sci.*, Vol. 99, No. 8, (August 2008), pp. 1501–1506, ISSN 1347-9032

Ostman, A. (2004). PDGF receptors-mediators of autocrine tumor growth and regulators of tumor vasculature and stroma. *Cytokine growth Factor Rev.*, Vol. 15, No. 4, (August 2004), pp. 275-286, ISSN 1359-6101

Oura, H., Bertoncini, J., Velasco, P., Brown, L. F., Carmeliet, P. & Detmar, M. (2003). A critical role of placenta growth factor in the induction of inflammation and edema formation. *Blood*, Vol. 101, No. 2, (January 2003), pp. 560-567, ISSN 0006-4971

Oyama, T., Ran, S., Ishida, T., Nadaf, S., Kerr, L., Carbone, D. P. & Gabrilovich, D. I. (1998). Vascular endothelial growth factor affects dendritic cell maturation through the inhibition of nuclear factor-kappa B activation in hemopoietic progenitor cells. *J Immunol.*, Vol. 160, No. 3, (February 1998), pp. 1224-1232, ISSN 0022-1767

Palumbo, C., Bei, R., Procopio, A. & Modesti A. (2008). Molecular targets and targeted therapies for malignant mesothelioma. *Curr. Med. Chem.*, Vol. 15, No. 9, pp. 855-867, ISSN 0929-8673

Parr, C., Watkins, G., Boulton, M., Cai, J. & Jiang, W. G. (2005). Placenta growth factor is over-expressed and has prognostic value in human breast cancer. *Eur. J. Cancer*, Vol. 41, No. 18, (December 2005), pp. 2819-2827, ISSN 0014-2964

Persico, M. G., Vincenti, V. & DiPalma, T. (1999). Structure, expression and receptor-binding properties of placenta growth factor (PlGF). *Curr. Top. Microbiol. Immunol.*, Vol. 237, pp. 31-40, ISSN 0070-217X

Philip, M., Rowley, D. A. & Schreiber, H. (2004). Inflammation as a tumor promoter in cancer induction. *Semin. Cancer Biol.*, Vol. 14, No. 6, (December 2004), pp. 433-439, ISSN 1044-579X

Pisick, E. & Salgia, R. (2005). Molecular biology of malignant mesothelioma: a review. *Hematol. Oncol. Clin. North Am.*, Vol. 19, No. 6, (December 2005), pp. 997-1023, ISSN 0889-8588

Plate, K. H., Breier, G., Millauer, B., Ullrich, A. & Risau, W. (1993). Up-regulation of vascular endothelial growth factor and its cognate receptors in a rat glioma model of tumor angiogenesis. *Cancer Res.*, Vol. 53, No., 23, (December 1993), pp. 5822-5827, ISSN 0008-5472

Pollard, J. W. (2004). Tumor-educated macrophages promote tumor progression and metastasis. *Nat. Rev. Cancer*, Vol. 4, No. 1, (January 2004), pp. 71–78, ISSN 1474, 175X

Pompeo, E., Albonici, L., Doldo, E., Orlandi, A., Manzari, V., Modesti, A. & Mineo, T. C. (2009). Placenta growth factor expression has prognostic value in malignant pleural mesothelioma. *Ann. Thorac. Surg.*, Vol. 88, No. 2, pp. 426-431, ISSN 0003-4975

Porta, C., Larghi, P., Rimoldi, M., Totaro, M. G., Allavena, P., Mantovani, A. & Sica, A. (2009). Cellular and molecular pathways linking inflammation and cancer. *Immunobiology*, Vol. 214, No. 9-10, pp. 761-777, ISSN 0171-2985

Rafii, S., Avecilla, S., Shmelkov, S., Shido, K., Tejada, R., Moore, M. A., Heissig, B. & Hattori, K. (2003). Angiogenic factors reconstitute hematopoiesis by recruiting stem cells from bone marrow microenvironment. *Ann. N. Y. Acad. Sci.*, Vol. 996, (May 2003), pp. 49-60, ISSN 0077-8923

Ramos-Ninos, M., Timblin, C. & Mossman, B. T. (2002). Mesothelial cell transformation requires increased AP-1 binding activity and ERK-dependent Fra-1 expression. *Cancer Res.*, Vol. 62, No. 21, (November 2002), pp. 6065-6069, ISSN 0008-5472

Reuter, S., Gupta, S. C., Chaturvedi, M. M. & Aggarwal, B. B. Oxidative stress, inflammation, and cancer: how are they linked? *Free Radic. Biol. Med.*, Vol. 49, No. 11, (December 2010), pp. 1603-1616, ISSN 0891-5849

Ribatti, D., Nico, B., Crivellato, E., Roccaro, A. M. & Vacca, A. (2007). The history of the angiogenic switch concept. *Leukemia*, Vol. 21, No. 1, (January 2007), pp. 44-52, ISSN 0887-6924

Riganti, C., Orecchia, S., Silvagno, F., Pescarmona, G., Betta, P. G., Gazzano, E., Aldieri, E., Ghigo, D. & Bosia A. (2007). Asbestos induces nitric oxide synthesis in mesothelioma cells via Rho signaling inhibition. *Am. J. Respir. Cell. Mol. Biol.*, Vol. 36, No. 6, (June 2007), pp. 746-756, ISSN 1044-1549

Robinson, B. W. & Lake, R. A. (2005). Advances in malignant mesothelioma. *N. Engl. J. Med.*, Vol. 353, No. 15, (October 2005), pp. 1591-1603, ISSN 0028-4793

Robledo, R. & Mossman, B. (1999). Cellular and molecular mechanisms of asbestos-induced fibrosis. *J. Cell. Physiol.*, Vol. 180, No. 2, (August 1999), pp. 158-166, ISSN 0021-9541

Roos, W. P. & Kaina, B. (2006). DNA damage-induced cell death by apoptosis. *Trends Mol. Med.*, Vol. 12, No. 9, (September 2006), pp. 440-450, ISSN 1471-4914

Rose-John, S., Waetzig, G. H., Scheller, J., Grötzinger, J. & Seegert, D. (2007). The IL-6/sIL-6R complex as a novel target for therapeutic approaches. *Expert Opin. Ther. Targets*, Vol. 11, No. 5, (May 2007), pp. 613-624, ISSN 1472-8222

Roskoski, R. Jr. (2007). Vascular endothelial growth factor (VEGF) signaling in tumor progression. *Crit. Rev. Oncol. Hematol.*, Vol. 62, No. 3, (June 2007), pp. 179-213, ISSN 1040-8428

Royds, J. A., Dower, S. K., Qwarnstrom, E. E. & Lewis, C. E. (1998). Response of tumour cells to hypoxia: role of p53 and NFkB. *Mol. Pathol.*, Vol. 51, No. 2, (April 1998), pp. 55-61, ISSN 1366-8714

Saccani, S., Pantano, S. & Natoli, G. (2003) Modulation of NF-kappaB activity by Exchange of dimers. *Mol. Cell*, Vol. 11, No. 6, (June 2003), pp. 1563-1574, ISSN 1097-2765

Saylor, P, J., Escudier, B. & Michaelson, M. D. (2012). Importance of Fibroblast Growth Factor Receptor in Neovascularization and Tumor Escape from Antiangiogenic Therapy. *Clin. Genitourin. Cancer*, (February 2012), Epub ahead of print, ISSN 1558-7673

Scheidereit, C. (2006). IkappaB kinase complexes: gateways to NF-kappaB activation and transcription. *Oncogene*, Vol. 25, No. 51, (2006), (October 2006), pp. 6685–6705, ISSN 0950-9232

Shaulian, E. & Karin, M. (2001). AP-1 in cell proliferation and survival. *Oncogene*, Vol. 20, No. 19, (April 2001), pp. 2390-2400, ISSN 0950-9232

Shaulian, E. & Karin, M. (2002). AP-1 as a regulator of cell life and death. *Nat. Cell Biol.*, Vol. 4, No. 5, (May 2002), pp. E131-E136, ISSN 1465-7392

Shaw, J. P., Utz, P. J., Durand, D. B., Toole, J. J., Emmel, E. A. & Crabtree, G. R. (1988). Identification of a putative regulator of early T cell activation genes. *Science*, Vol. 241, No. 4862, (July 1988), pp. 202–205, ISSN 0036-8075

Shibuya, M. (2006). Differential roles of vascular endothelial growth factor receptor-1 and receptor-2 in angiogenesis. *J. Biochem. Mol. Biol.*, Vol. 39, No. 5, (September 2006), pp. 469-478, ISSN 1225-8687

Schonthaler, H. B., Guinea-Viniegra, J. & Wagner, E. F. (2011). Targeting inflammation by modulating the Jun/AP-1 pathway. *Ann. Rheum, Dis.*, Vol. 70, Suppl. 1, (March 2011), pp. i109-i112, ISSN 0003-4967

Shukla, A., Gulumian, M., Hei, T. K., Kamp, D., Rahman, Q. & Mossman, B. T. (2003a). Multiple roles of oxidants in the pathogenesis of asbestos-induced diseases. *Free Radical Biol. Med.*, Vol. 34, No. 9, (May 2003), pp. 1117–1129, ISSN 0891-5849

Shukla, A., Jung, M., Stern, M., Fukagawa, N. K., Taatjes, D. J., Sawyer, D., Van Houte,n B. & Mossman B. T. (2003b). Asbestos induces mitochondrial DNA damage and dysfunction linked to the development of apoptosis. *Am. J. Physiol. Lung Cell. Mol. Physiol.*, Vol. 285, No. 5, (November 2003), pp. L1018–L1025, ISSN 1040-0605

Sica, A. (2010). Role of tumour-associated macrophages in cancer-related inflammation. *Exp. Oncol.*, Vol. 32, No. 3, (September 2010), pp. 153-158, ISSN 1812-9269

Simeonova, P. & Luster, M. (1995). Iron and reactive oxygen species in the asbestos-induced tumor necrosis factor-α response from alveolar macrophages. *Am. J. Respir. Cell. Mol. Biol.*, Vol. 12, No. 6, (June 1995), pp. 676–683, ISSN 1044-1549

Simeonova, P. P., Toriumi, W., Kommineni, C., Erkan, M., Munson, A. E., Rom, W. N. & Luster, M. I. (1997). Molecular regulation of IL-6 activation by asbestos in lung epithelial cells: role of reactive oxygen species. *J. Immunol.*, Vol. 159, No. 8, (October 1997), pp. 3921-3928, ISSN 0022-1767

Stapelberg, M., Gellert, N., Swettenham, E., Tomasetti, M., Witting, P. K., Procopio, A. & Neuzil, J. (2005). Alpha-tocopheryl succinate inhibits malignant mesothelioma by disrupting the fibroblast growth factor autocrine loop: mechanism and the role of oxidative stress. *J. Biol. Chem.*, Vol. 280, No. 27, (July 2005), pp. 25369-25376, ISSN 0021-9258

Strizzi, L., Catalano, A., Vianale, G., Orecchia, S., Casalini, A., Tassi, G., Puntoni, R., Mutti, L. & Procopio, A. (2001a). Vascular endothelial growth factor is an autocrine growth factor in human malignant mesothelioma. *J. Pathol.*, Vol. 193, No. 4. (April 2001), pp. 468-475, ISSN 0022-3417

Strizzi, L., Vianale, G., Catalano,. A., Muraro, R., Mutti, L. & Procopio, A. (2001b). Basic fibroblast growth factor in mesothelioma pleural effusions: correlation with patient survival and angiogenesis. *Int. J. Oncol.*, Vol. 18, No. 5, (May 2001), pp. 1093-1098, ISSN 1019-6439

Sun, S. C. (2011). Non-canonical NF-κB signaling pathway. *Cell Res.*, Vol. 21, No. 1, (January 2011), pp. 71-85, ISSN 1001-0602

Takahashi, A., Kono, K., Ichihara, F., Sugai, H., Fuji, H. & Matsumoto, Y. (2004).Vascular endothelial growth factor inhibits maturation of dendritic cells induced by lipopolysaccharide, but not by proinflammatory cytokines. *Cancer Immunol., Immunother.*, Vol. 53, No. 6, (June 2004), pp. 543-550, ISSN 0340-7004

Tanaka, S., Choe, N., Hemenway, D. R., Zhu, S., Matalon, S. & Kagan, E. (1998). Asbestos inhalation induces reactive nitrogen species and nitrotyrosine formation in the lungs and pleura of the rat. *J. Clin. Invest.*, Vol. 102, No. 2, (July 1998), pp. 445–454, ISSN 0021-9738

Toi, M., Matsumoto, T. & Bando, H. (2001). Vascular endothelial growth factor: its prognostic, predictive, and therapeutic implications. *Lancet Oncol.*, Vol. 2, No. 11, (November 2001), pp. 667-673, ISSN 1470-2045

Toyokuni, S. (2009). Mechanisms of asbestos-induced carcinogenesis. *Nagoya J. Med. Sci.*, Vol. 71, No. 1-2, (February 2009), pp. 1-10, ISSN 0027-7622

Toyooka, S., Kishimoto, T. & Date, H. (2008). Advances in the molecular biology of malignant mesothelioma. *Acta Med., Okayama,* Vol. 62, No. 1, (February 2008), pp. 1-7, ISSN 0386-300X

Ullrich, E., Bonmort, M., Mignot, G., Kroemer, G. & Zitvogel, L. (2008). Tumor stress, cell death and the ensuing immune response. *Cell Death Differ.,* Vol. 15, No. 1, (January 2008), pp. 21-28, ISSN 1350-9047

Valle, M. T., Castagneto, B., Procopio, A., Carbone, M., Giordano, A. & Mutti, L. (1998). Immunobiology and immune defense mechanisms of mesothelioma cells. *Monaldi Arch. Chest Dis.*, Vol. 53, No. 2, (April 1998), pp. 219-227, ISSN 1122-0643

Villanova, F., Procopio, A. & Rippo, M. R. (2008). Malignant mesothelioma resistance to apoptosis: recent discoveries and their implication for effective therapeutic strategies. *Curr. Med. Chem.*, Vol. 15, No. 7, pp. 631-641, ISSN 0929-8673

Waltenberger, J., Claesson-Welsh, L., Siegbahn, A., Shibuya, M. & Heldin, C. H. (1994). Different signal transduction properties of KDR and Flt1, two receptors for vascular endothelial growth factor. *J. Biol. Chem.*, Vol. 269, No. 43, (October 1994), pp. 26988-26995, ISSN 0021-9258

Wei, S. C., Tsao, P. N., Yu, S. C., Shun, C. T., Tsai-Wu, J. J., Wu, C. H., Su, Y. N., Hsieh, F. J. & Wong, J. M. (2005). Placenta growth factor expression is correlated with survival of patients with colorectal cancer. *Gut*, Vol. 54, No. 5, (May 2005), pp. 666-672, ISSN 0017-5749

Wu, W. S. (2006). The signaling mechanism of ROS in tumor progression. *Cancer Metastasis Rev.*, Vol. 25, No. 4, (December 2006), pp. 695-705, ISSN 0167-7659

Yang, H., Bocchetta, M., Kroczynska, B., Elmishad, A. G., Chen, Y., Liu, Z., Bubici, C., Mossman, B. T., Pass, H. I., Testa, J. R., Franzoso, G. & Carbone, M. (2006). TNF-alpha inhibits asbestos-induced cytotoxicity via a NF-kappaB-dependent pathway, a possible mechanism for asbestos-induced oncogenesis. *Proc. Natl. Acad. Sci. USA.,* Vol. 103, No. 27, (July 2006), pp. 10397–10402, ISSN 0027-8424

Yarborough, C.M. (2007). The risk of mesothelioma from exposure to chrysotile asbestos. Curr. Opin. Pulm. Med., Vol. 13, No. 4, (July 2007), pp. 334-338, ISSN 1070-5287

Yasumitsu, A., Tabata, C., Tabata, R., Hirayama, N., Murakami, A., Yamada, S., Terada, T., Iida, S., Tamura, K., Fukuoka, K., Kuribayashi, K. & Nakano, T. (2010). Clinical significance of serum vascular endothelial growth factor in malignant pleural mesothelioma. *J. Thorac. Oncol.*, Vol. 5, No. 4, (April 2010), pp. 479-483, ISSN 1556-0864

Yoo, S. A., Kwok, S. K. & Kim W. U. (2008). Proinflammatory role of vascular endothelial growth factor in the pathogenesis of rheumatoid arthritid: prospect for therapeutic intervention. *Mediators Inflamm.*, Vol. 2008, Article ID 129873, ISSN 0962-9351

Yoshida, K. & Miki, Y. (2010). The cell death machinery governed by the p53 tumor suppressor in response to DNA damage. *Cancer Sci.*, Vol. 101, No. 4, (April 2010), pp. 831-835, ISSN 1347-9032

Zebrowski, B. K., Yano, S., Liu, W., Shaheen, R. M., Hicklin, D. J., Putnam, J. B. & Ellis, L. M. (1999). Vascular endothelial growth factor levels and induction of permeability in malignant pleural effusions. *Clin. Cancer Res.*, Vol. 5, No. 11, (November 1999), pp. 3364-3368, ISSN 1078-0432

Ziogas, A. C., Gavalas, N. G., Tsiatas, M., Tsitsilonis, O., Politi, E., Terpos, E., Rodolakis, A., Vlahos, G., Thomakos, N., Haidopoulos, D., Antsaklis, A., Dimopoulos, M. A. & Bamias, A. (2012). VEGF directly suppresses activation of T cells from ovarian cancer patients and healthy individuals via VEGF receptor Type 2. *Int. J. Cancer.*, Vol. 130, No. 4, (February 2012), pp. 857-864, ISSN 0020-7136

Chapter 4

The Role of Cyclooxygenase-2, Epidermal Growth Factor Receptor and Aromatase in Malignant Mesothelioma

Rossella Galati

Additional information is available at the end of the chapter

http://dx.doi.org/10.5772/50674

1. Introduction

Malignant mesothelioma (MM) is a rare malignant disease originating from neoplastic mesothelial cells which compose the serous membranes of pleura, peritoneum, pericardium, or testis. Mesothelioma responds little to chemo and radiotherapy and is associated with a poor prognosis. In Western Europe, the incidence is increasing and is expected to peak in the year 2020 (Peto et al., 1999; Pelucchi et al., 2004) while in Japan and Australia, the peak is expected for 2025 and 2015 respectively. Thus in order to improve the clinical outcome in the pharmacological treatment of this refractory tumour, drugs directed against novel and/or characterized tumour-specific cellular targets are needed. Malignant pleural mesothelioma (MPM) originates from the pleural layers. Pleura is not just a limiting protective layer for lung, but a dynamic cellular structure regulating serial responses to injury, infection, and disease. Mesothelial cells are biologically active because they can sense and respond to signals within their microenvironment. The development of MM is associated in most patients with a history of asbestos exposure (Mossman et al., 1996). In addition, some investigations have implicated SV40 virus in the pathogenesis of a subset of mesotheliomas (Carbone et al., 2003). Exposure to asbestos typically occurs during mining and milling of the fibers or during industrial application of asbestos in textiles, insulation, shipbuilding, brake lining mechanics, and other areas. Non occupational exposure is usually related to asbestos fibers inadvertently released into the environment and transported by asbestos-contaminated clothing or other materials. After asbestos inhalation, fibers deposited in the lungs typically remain in close contact with lung epithelial cells. Since this fiber-cell interaction could potentially initiate or inhibit cellular functions, asbestos acts as a carcinogen by initiating the carcinogenic process. Carcinogens are known to modulate the transcription factors, anti-apoptotic proteins, proapoptotic proteins, protein kinases, cell cycle proteins, cell adhesion molecules, cyclooxygenase-2, and growth factor signaling pathways. Research has demonstrated that asbestos exposure generates reactive oxygen species and activates macrophages and other cell types to produce these compounds as well as cytokines and growth factors (Kamp & Weitzman, 1999). Furthermore, the deposition of insoluble amphibole fibers results in a chronic inflammatory state and increased rates of MM in exposed individuals (Mossman & Churg, 1998). This article reviews recent studies regarding some MM molecular targets involved in inflammation for not only prevention but also for therapy of this deadly cancer.

2. MM molecular targets involved in inflammation

The existence of inflammation has been associated with up-regulation of the inducible cyclooxygenases-2 (COX-2), leading to an increase in its product prostaglandin-E2 (PGE-2) (Vane et al., 1994), and is associated with an increased risk of cancer (Ambs et al., 1999). Considerable evidence indicates that COX-2–derived PGE2 can activate epidermal growth factor receptor (EGFR) signaling and thereby stimulate cell proliferation. The mechanism(s) by which this occurs seem to be complex and context specific. Regardless of the precise mechanism for doing so, exposure to COX-2–derived PGE2 can initiate a positive feedback loop whereby activation of EGFR results in enhanced expression of COX-2 and increased synthesis of prostaglandins (Lippman et al., 2005). Although there is a crosstalk between EGFR and COX-2 in carcinogenesis it is important to stress that EGFR and its downstream effectors can be activated independently of COX-2/PGE2. For example, in MM, asbestos fibers activate the EGFR resulting in activation of extracellular signal regulated kinase downstream (Shukla et al., 2011). Similarly, COX-2/PGE2 and its downstream effectors can be regulated independently of EGFR signaling. For example, PGE2 is able to rapidly stimulate Erk phosphorylation in a subset of non–small cell lung cancer (NSCLC) cell lines via intracellular activation of kinase cascades independently of the proteolytic release of EGFR ligands via Src. (Gutkind, 1998; Krysan et al., 2005). These findings have provided the underpinnings for developing agents targeting EGFR or COX-2. A recent study with COX-2 and EGFR inhibitors in MM has shown that the differences in the susceptibility to drugs could be due to the differences in the signalling pathways affected, in addition to the responses that may depend on cell type. In particular it was demonstrated in the Ist-Mes-2 MM cell line a synergistic effect on the inhibition of cell growth between the active small molecule inhibitor of EGFR, gefitinib and rofecoxib, a drug that specifically targets COX-2. Interestingly, the other two cell lines sensitive to treatment with single drugs Ist-Mes-1 and MPP89, did not display this synergistic effect. Only in Ist-Mes-2, the cell line where p-AKT was not detectable, did the combination of rofecoxib and gefitinib result in a synergistic effect. This study suggests that identifying the mechanisms that underlie these differences in sensitivity of cell lines of MM single agents and their combinations, can help us to explore new proteins involved in drug resistance. (Stoppoloni et al., 2010). Lately a new therapeutic target, the Aromatase (CYP19A1), has been identified in MM. This new discovery has highlighted the possibility that there may be in MM as well as in breast cancer a relationship between inflammation, COX-2, EGFR and Aromatase (Fig.1)(Chumsri et al. 2011. These key molecules and pathways that connect chronic inflammation with inflammation associated oncogenic transformation will be described. We emphasize how the increased understanding of the role of COX-2, EGFR and CYP19A1 in MM may provide novel preventive, diagnostic and therapeutic strategies for MM.

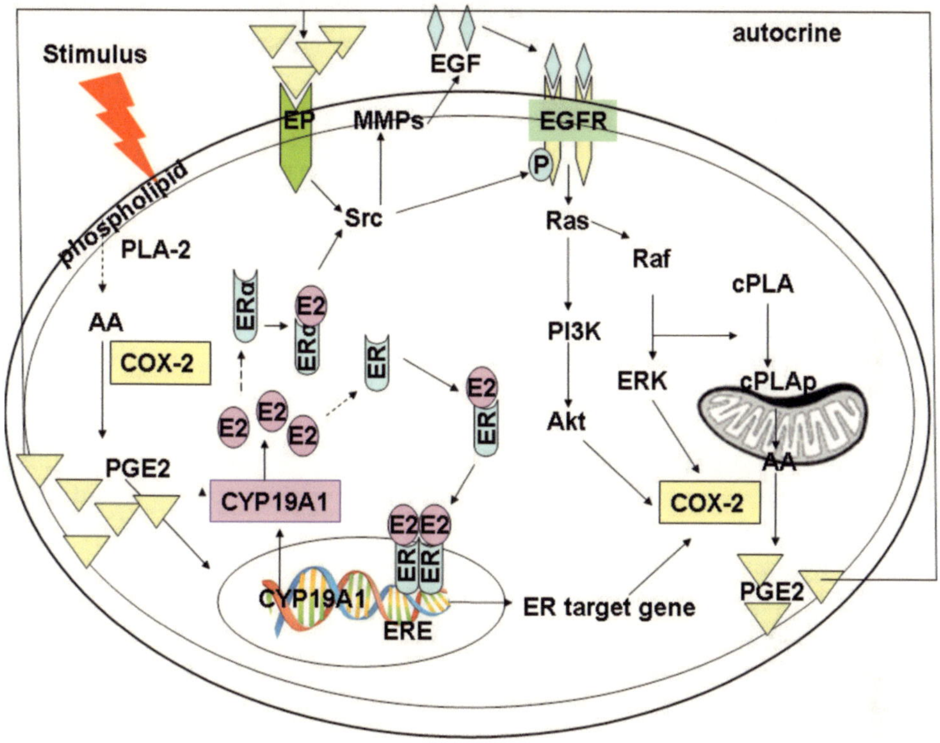

Figure 1. Posible relationship among inflammation, COX-2, EGFR and Aromatase.

Arachidonic acid (AA) metabolic pathway can be activated by inflammation (Stimulus). AA is released from membrane phospholipids by a phospholipase named phospholipase A2 (PLA-2) enzyme and converted to bioactive PGE-2 by COX-2. PGE_2 is an important regulator of *CYP19A1* gene expression and stimulates CYP19A1 activity to increase localized estrogen 17-beta-estradiol (E2). The E2 binds to the classical estrogen receptor (ER) to promote its dimerization and translocation to the nucleus where it modulates the expression of estrogen target genes (COX-2). The interaction of E_2 with ER-alpha also activates signaling cascades that promote cell proliferation, such as the activation of of c-Src tyrosine kinase (Src). Src can also be activated by binding of PGE2 to its receptor (EP). Src activation induces the EGFR phosphorilation and stimulates the matrix metalloproteinase cascade which culminates in the liberation of epidermal growth factor (EGF). Free EGF ligand binds to EGFR family receptors that activates extracellular-signal-regulate- kinase (ERK). Cytosolic phospholipase A_2 (cPLA) is a substrate for ERK and phosphorylation of cPLA (cPLAp) promotes its association with intracellular membranes such as those of the endoplasmic reticulum and mitochondria and releases lysophospholipids and AA from these membranes. COX-2 catalyses the conversion of AA into PGE-2.

2.1. Cyclooxygenases

COXs, also known as prostaglandin-endoperoxide synthases, are key regulatory enzymes in the biosynthesis of prostanoids, a class of hormones including prostaglandins, prostacyclins, and thromboxanes responsible for multiple inflammatory mitogenic, and angiogenic activities in various tissue and organ systems. Increasing interest on COXs is due to the many evidences showing the involvement of these enzymes not only in physiologic but even in pathophysiologic processes such as development and progression of cancer. Two COX isoforms have been identified as COX-1 and COX-2. COX-1 is expressed constitutively in several cell types of normal mammalian tissues, where it is involved in the maintenance of tissue homeostasis. In contrast, COX-2 is an inducible enzyme responsible for PGE2 production at sites of inflammation (Harris, 2007). The mechanism through which COX-2 exherts its tumorigenic action can be directly mediated by the enzyme or due to effects of its products. COX-2 is an oxygenase and its intermediates are highly reactive. It is possible that these compounds may cause free radical damage, for example, against DNA molecule (Cardillo et al., 2005) . There is considerable evidence that prostaglandins, participate both in normal growth responses and in aberrant growth, including carcinogenesis (Greenhough et al., 2009). PGE2 exerts its autocrine/paracrine effects on target cells by binding to four types of membrane-bound, G protein-coupled receptors termed as EP1, EP2, EP3, and EP4 (E-series prostanoid receptors) (Narumiya et al. 1999). These receptors are often coexpressed in the same cell type and use different, and in some cases, opposing intracellular signalling pathways (Breyer et al. 2001).Following ligand binding, the EP receptors activate different signal transduction pathways. EP1 raises intracellular Ca2_, whereas EP3 reduces or increases cyclic -adenosin monophosphate (cAMP) by activating inhibitory G (Gi) or stimulatory G (Gs) proteins depending on the particular splice variant expressed by the cell (Kotani, M et al. 1995). The EP2 and EP4 receptors increase intracellular cAMP by activating adenylate cyclase via Gs proteins. However, differences in the strength of Gs coupling, activation of other signal transduction pathways, agonist-induced desensitization, and agonist-induced internalization result in a differential response of the target cell to a ligand-induced activation of the EP2 or EP4 receptors (Akaogi et al. 2006).It was shown that PGE2 stimulation of both EP2 and EP4 receptors involves transactivation of the epidermal growth factor receptor (EGFR) signaling pathway to promote tumorigenesis (Buchanan et al.; Pai et al 2003; Sale set al. 2005). PGE-2 promotes tumor growth with subsequent enhancement of cellular proliferation, promotion and angiogenesis, stimulation of invasion/mobility, suppression of immune responses and inhibitiuon of programmed cell death by inducing expression of the Bcl-2 protooncogene (which can suppress apoptosis) (Cardillo et al.,2005) (Fig.2).

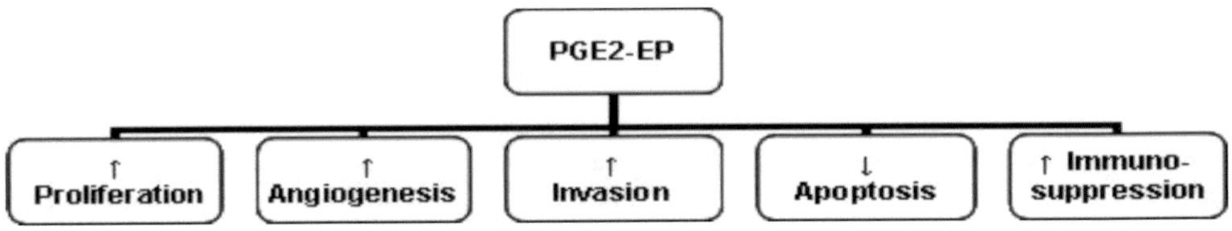

Figure 2. PGE2 in carcinogenesis

For several types of cancer the real risk factor seems to be chronic inflammation (Prescott & Fitzpatrick, 2000) that maintains high level of COX-2 and increase events that promote tumor formation. A tragic example of this mechanism is MM. Although molecular mechanisms of asbestos tumorigenicity have not been elucidated, research has shown that deposition of insoluble amphibole fibers results in a chronic inflammatory state (Mossman & Churg, 1998) and that this state generates reactive oxygen and nitrogen species, as well as cytokines and growth factors, through the activation of macrophages and other cell types (Kamp & Weitzman, 1999).

As expected, the prolonged inflammation causes the increase of COX-2 level, that is actually recognized as an important MM prognostic factor (Edwards et al., 2002; Mineo et al., 2010). A study clearly demonstrated that COX-2 expression is a strong prognostic factor in human mesothelioma, which contributes independently to the other clinical and histopathologic factors in determining a short survival (Edwards et al., 2002). Although the regulation of mRNA stability appears to be the most important regulatory step for COX-2 expression, several studies have reported that other mechanisms, such as transcriptional control or hypermethylation (Dixon et al., 2000), also are involved in the regulation of COX-2 expression. In cancer cells, it was demonstrated previously that altered post-transcriptional regulation of COX-2 is mediated by increased cytoplasmic mRNA binding of the mRNA stability factor HuR (Dixon et al., 2001). In MM, the cytoplasmic expression of HuR was correlated significantly with high COX-2 expression and with poor survival (Stoppoloni et al.,2008). Finally, COX-2 has been proposed to exert its influence on mesangial cell proliferation *in vitro* by a novel mechanism involving the tumor suppressor p53 and the cell cycle inhibitors p21 and p27 (Zahner et al., 2002). Interestingly, several studies have investigated the potential prognostic value of p53, p21 and p27 in malignant mesotheliomas, thus reinforcing the evidence of a primary role of COX-2 in the pathogenesis and progression of MM (Bongiovanni et al., 2001; Baldi et al., 2002). Due to the lack of a reliable treatment capable of achieving long-term control in mesothelioma patients, these enzymes are becoming more and more appealing as potential therapeutic targets (Veltman et al., 2010; Stoppoloni et al., 2010; O'Kane et al., 2010)

2.2. Epidermal growth factor receptor

The epidermal growth factor receptor (EGFR) is the cell-surface receptor for members of the epidermal growth factor family (EGF-family) of extracellular protein ligands (Herbst, 2004). Upon activation by its growth factor ligands, EGFR undergoes a transition from an inactive monomeric form to an active homodimer. In addition, EGFR may pair with another member of the ErbB receptor family, such as ErbB2/Her2/neu, to create an activated heterodimer. EGFR dimerization stimulates its intrinsic intracellular protein-tyrosine kinase activity. As a result, autophosphorylation of several tyrosine residues in the C-terminal domain of EGFR occurs (P-EGFR). This autophosphorylation leads to the activation of downstream signalling cascades including the RAS/extracellular signal regulated kinase (ERK) pathway, the phosphatidylinositol 3-kinase/AKT (PI3K/AKT) pathway and the Janus kinase/Signal transducer and activator of transcription (JAK/ STAT) pathway (Fig.3).

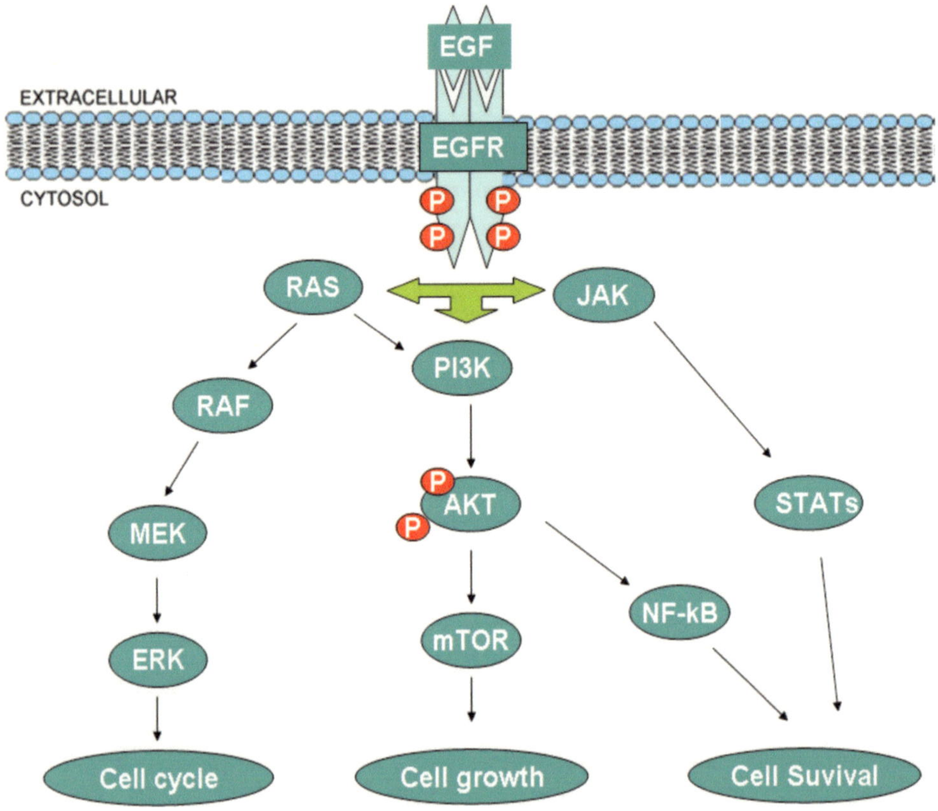

Figure 3. Activation of downstream signaling cascade by P-EGFR

These pathways act in a coordinated manner to promote cell survival (Oda et al., 2005). Such proteins modulate phenotypes such as cell migration, adhesion, and proliferation. EGFR is reportedly over-expressed in a wide variety of malignancies. Various studies suggest that receptor tyrosine kinase activation participates in the oncogenic progression of non neoplastic mesothelial progenitor cells to malignant mesothelioma. Asbestos fiber interact with the external domain of the EGFR to cause dimerization, activation and increased EGFR mRNA and protein levels in rat and human SV-40 immortalized mesothelial cells (Shukla et al., 2011). Up-regulated EGFR and resulting tyrosine phosphorylation leads to the Ras activation which phosphorylates directly and activates Raf (Rapidly Accelerated Fibrosarcoma). Raf is responsible for phosphorylation of the mitogen associated / extracellular regulated kinase-1 (MEK) which in turn phosphorylates extracellular regulated kinases (ERK) on specific residues of threonine and tyrosine (Ras-Raf-MEK-ERK mitogen activated protein kinase (MAPK) pathway). ERK activates a variety of substrates involved in cell cycle. The ERK family consists of at least seven isoforms, and little is known about their regulation and function. ERK1/2 phosphorylation by asbestos, is dependent on phosphorylation of the EGFR. Moreover, has been shown that ERK5, a redox-sensitive kinase known to mediate c-*jun* proto-oncogene expression is activated by asbestos. ERK1/2 and ERK5 are all important in asbestos-induced proliferation and this may be the result of increases in the mRNA levels of AP-1 family members. The ERK5 pathway may be contributing selectively to the regulation of c-*jun*, whereas ERK1/2 pathways may regulate c-*fos*, *fra*-1 and c-*jun*. Has been linked ERK1/2-dependent *fra*-1 expression to mesothelial cell transformation by asbestos and the protracted expression of this gene may be a result of initial increases in c-*fos* and c-*jun* (Scapoli et al., 2004). The phosphoinositide 3-kinase (PI3K)/AKT pathway, plays a critical role for the cell cycle progression in human MM cells [Altomare et al.,2005). AKT, and the downstream mTOR are involved in cell growth and survival, and they are often found to be activated in MM (Carbone et al., 2012). It was reported previously that STAT1 and STAT3 are deregulated MM (Kothmaier et al., 2008).The JAK/STAT signalling pathway is the principal signalling mechanism for growth factors in mammals. JAK activation induces a variety of biological responses such as cell proliferation, diff erentiation and cell migration. In addition, MM cell lines are reported to express EGFR and transforming growth factor-α (TGF-α), suggesting an autocrine role for EGFR in MM (Cai et al., 2004; Jänne et al., 2002). EGFR immunopositivity has been indicated as a poor prognostic factor in many solid tumors in the past (Nicholson et al., 2001). The EGFR expression in MM has been previously reported, with controversial results, possibly due to the lack of standardized method for EGFR detection and quantification (Dazzi et al., Destro et al., 2006; 1990; Govindan et al., 2005; Ramael et al., 1991; Trupiano et al., 2004). Until now, the role of immunohistochemistry (IHC) EGFR positive staining in influencing prognosis of MM is not clear. Some authors did not find differences in survival when IHC EGFR positive or negative staining were compared (Destro et al., 2006; Okuda et al., 2008). This is because only few reports analyzed the effect of IHC EGFR positive status and cell subtype in MM patients. Recently EGFR overexpression is identified by IHC in 52% of epithelial MM and is demonstrated to be a factor negatively affecting prognosis (Rena et al., 2011). In view of these studies, EGFR was targeted for MM therapy, but despite the high expression of EGFR not all cells are sensitive to EGFR inhibitors (Garland et al., 2007). Many efforts are now directed to understand the lack of sensitivity of MM to EGFR inhibitors. In one such study, EGFR mutations were found in 31% (9 of 29) of malignant mesothelioma cases. Seven of these mutations were novel, and one was the L858R mutation described in NSCLC (Foster et al., 2009). Activating EGFR mutations in MM associated with optimal resectability and prolonged survival. Clinically these mutations may ultimately have utility in patient selection for surgery, systemic therapy, and selection for EGFR-TKI (tyrosine kinase inhibitor). The clinical course of MM patients with EGFR mutant tumors appear to share same 'relative' improved clinical outcome like mutant EGFR-NSCLC (Foster et al., 2010 . Study shows the ineffectiveness of the EGFR inhibitors due to coactivation of multiple receptor tyrosine kinase (EGFR, ERBB3, MET, and AXL) in individual mesothelioma cell lines (Ou et al., 2011) Thus, a combination therapy, could be a winning strategy in the treatment of mesothelioma.

2.3. Aromatase

A novel marker of MM recently identified is the CYP19A1 (Stoppoloni et al., 2011). CYP19A1 is the cytochrome P450 enzyme complex that converts C19 androgens to C18 estrogens. The human CYP19A1 gene, located in the 21.2 region on the long arm of chromosome 15 (15q21.2), spans a region that consists of a 30 kb coding region and a 93 kb regulatory region. Its regulatory region contains at least 10 distinct promoters regulated in a tissue- or signalling pathway-specific manner. Each promoter is regulated by a distinct set of regulatory sequences in DNA and transcription factors that bind to these specific sequences. These partially tissue-specific promoters are used in the gonads, bone, brain, vascular tissue, adipose tissue, skin, foetal liver, and placenta for estrogen biosynthesis necessary for human physiology (Bulun et al., 2004). Estrogens contribute to differentiation and maturation in normal lung (Patrone et al., 2003) and also stimulate growth and progression of lung tumors (Stabile et al., 2002; Pietras et al., 2005). Two major pathways, generally termed genomic and non-genomic, are known to mediate estradiol effects on cells. (Fig.4)

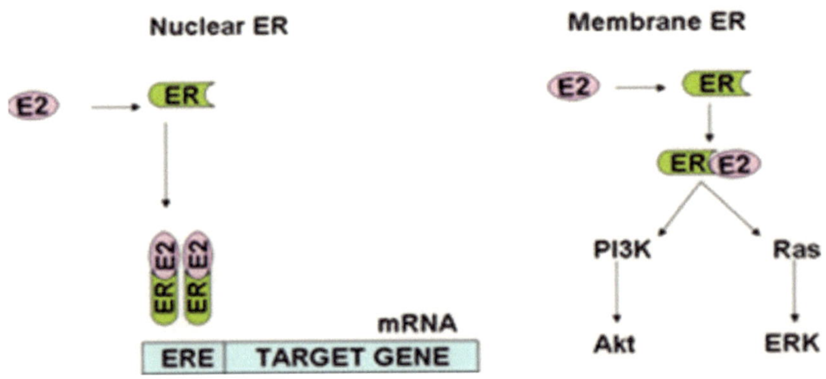

Figure 4. Estrogen Receptor fuction: Genomic (Nuclear ER) and Non Genomic (Membrane ER) action

Estradiol has traditionally been described to mediate its effects via intracellular receptors located in the cytoplasm or on the nuclear membrane and thus studies have investigated the effect of estradiol on transcription factors in the regulation of target genes . Estradiol also acts on the plasma membrane to initiate signaling pathways in the cytoplasm and regulate cellular functions, which is called the non-genomic pathway (Simoncini et al., 2004; Simoncini & Genazzani, 2003). PGE2 is thought to be an important regulator of CYP19A1 gene expression (Zhao et al., 1996). PGE2 increased CYP19A1 activity level in MM cell lines (Stoppoloni et al., 2011). Over the last decade many studies have been carried out to identify potential CYP19A1 stimulatory factors: IL-6 was the most potent factor detected that could stimulate CYP19A1 activity (Reed et al., 1992). The MM cell lines were capable of releasing a constitutively high amount of IL-6 (>1,100 pg.mL supernatant-1 of confluent cultures) (Orengo et al., 1999). This could explain the presence of CYP19A1 in MM cells. Furthermore, estrogen receptor (ER) were also detected in MM cell lines by western blot. The classic 67 kDa and a variant 46 kDa of ERα and 59 kDa of ERβ were expressed in MM cell lines. In support of these results there are recent literature data pointing to a role for estrogens in MM pathogenesis. Epidemiologic studies have identified female gender as a positive prognostic factor for MM (Pinton et al., 2009), although no experimental explanation of this finding has been provided thus far. CYP19A1 was expressed in the majority of samples from patients with MM. Cytoplasmic expression of CYP19A1 significantly correlated with poor survival (Stoppoloni et al., 2011). The World Health Organization classifies MM into epithelial, sarcomatoid, and biphasic types, each of which can be subdivided further (Travis et al., 1999). This classification has implications for both diagnosis and prognosis. Prognosis is poor for all MMs, but sarcomatoid MMs have a particularly poor response rate to treatment (Neragi-Miandoab et al., 2008). A significant association between high expression of CYP19A1 and sarcomatoid MMs was found (Stoppoloni et al., 2011). These observations strongly suggest that CYP19A1 plays a role in tumour progression in MM. MM cell proliferation was significantly reduced by exemestane (aromatase inhibitor) treatment. Treatment of MM cells with exemestane led to significant reduction of tumor cell growth, perturbation of cell cycle, caspase activation, PARP cleavage, down-regulation of p-AKT and Bcl-xL. . Since Akt pathway as well as Bcl-xL are implicated in conferring resistance to conventional chemotherapy exemestane could open new treatment strategies to be associated with standard therapy for patients afflicted with MM (Stoppoloni et al., 2011).

3. Conclusion

COX-2, EGFR and CYP19A1 are investigational at the present time. The cross-talk between markers that have been described and their value as prognostic indicators will need to be validated in prospective studies in larger patient populations. Their role at the present time is to give us direction towards development of newer therapies in this very resistant tumor. The standard of care at the present time for malignant mesothelioma does not involve checking for these markers and making patient care decisions based on them. But we hope that in the near future this would become a reality with a better treatment approach and prognosis for these patients. Furthermore the possibility of using natural anti-inflammatory products in the chemoprevention of people at risk of MM can not exclude.

Author details

Rossella Galati
Regina Elena Cancer Institute, Rome, Italy

4. References

Akaogi, J.; Nozaki, T.; Satoh. M.; & Yamada, H. (2006) Role of PGE2 and EP receptors in the pathogenesis of rheumatoid arthritis and as a novel therapeutic strategy. *Endocr Metab Immune Disord Drug Targets* 6,383–394.

Altomare, DA.; You, H.; Xiao,GH.; Ramos-Nino, ME.; Skele, KL.; De Rienzo, A.; Jhanwar, SC.; Mossman, BT.; Kane, AB.; Testa JR.(2005) Human and mouse mesotheliomas exhibit elevated AKT/PKB activity, which can be targeted pharmacologically to inhibit tumor cell growth. *Oncogene* 24,6080-6089.

Ambs, S.; Hussain, SP.; Marrogi, AJ. & Harris, CC. (1999). Cancer-prone oxyradical overload disease. *IARC Sci Publ*, 150,295-302.

Baldi, A.; Groeger, A.M.; Esposito, V.; Cassandro, R.; Tonini, G.; Battista, T.; Di Marino, MP.; Vincenzi, B.; Santini, M.; Angelini, A.; Rossiello, R.; Baldi F.& Paggi MG. (2002). Expression of p21 in SV40 large T antigen positive human pleural mesothelioma: relationship with survival. *Thorax*, 57,353-356

Bongiovanni, M.; Cassoni, P.; De Giuli, P.; Viberti, L.; Cappia, S.; Ivaldi, C.; Chiusa, L. & Bussolati, G. (2001). p27kip1 immunoreactivity correlates with long-term survival in pleural malignant mesothelioma. *Cancer*, 92,1245-1250

Breyer, RM.; Bagdassarian, CK.;Myers, SA. & Breyer, MD. (2001) Prostanoid receptors: subtypes and signalling. *Annu Rev Pharmacol Toxicol.* 41, 561–690

Buchanan, FG.; Wang, D.; Bargiacchi, F. & DuBois, RN. (2003) Prostaglandin E2 regulates cell migration via the intracellular activation of the epidermal growth factor receptor. *J Biol Chem* 278, 35451–35457

Bulun, SE.; Takayama, K.; Suzuki, T.; Sasano, H.; Yilmaz, B. & Sebastian, S. (2004). Organization of the human aromatase p450 (CYP19A1) gene. *Semin Reprod Med*, 22,5-9.

Cai, YC.; Roggli, V.; Mark, E.; Cagle, PT. & Fraire, AE. (2004). Transforming growth factor alpha and epidermal growth factor receptor in reactive and malignant mesothelial proliferations. *Arch Pathol Lab Med.*, 128,68–70.

Carbone, M.; Pass, HI.; Miele, L. & Bocchetta, M. (2003). New developments about the association of SV40 with human mesothelioma. *Oncogene*, 22,5173–5180

Carbone, M.; Yang, H. (2012) Molecular pathways: targeting mechanisms of asbestos and erionite carcinogenesis in mesothelioma. *Clin Cancer Res.*18,598-604.

Cardillo, I.; Spugnini, EP.; Verdina, A.; Galati, R.; Citro, G. & Baldi, A. (2005). Cox and mesothelioma, an overview. *Histol Histopathol*, 20,1267-1274

Chumsri, S.; Howes, T.; Bao, T.; Sabnis, G. & Brodie, A. (2011). Aromatase, aromatase inhibitors, and breast cancer. *J Steroid Biochem Mol Biol, 125,13-22*

Dazzi, H.; Hasleton, PS.; Thatcher, N.; Wilkes, S.; Swindell, R. & Chatterjee, AK. (1990) Malignant pleural mesothelioma and epidermal growth factor receptor (EGF-R). Relationship of EGF-R with histology and survival using fixed paraffin embedded tissue and the F4, monoclonal antibody. *Br J Cancer*, 61,924–926.

Destro, A.; Ceresoli, GL.; Falleni, M.; Zucali, PA.; Morenghi, E.; Bianchi, P.; Pellegrini, C.; Cordani, N.; Vaira, V.; Alloisio, M.; Rizzi, A.; Bosari, S. &, Roncalli, M. (2006). EGFR overexpression in malignant pleural mesothelioma. An immunohistochemical and molecular study with clinico-pathological correlations. *Lung Cancer*, 51,207–215.

Dixon, DA.; Kaplan, CD.; McIntyre, TM.; Zimmerman, GA. & Prescott, SM. (2000). Post-transcriptional control of cyclooxygenase-2 gene expression. The role of the 30-untranslated region. *J Biol Chem.*, 275,11750-11757

Dixon, DA.; Tolley, ND.; King, PH.; Nabors, LB.; McIntyre, TM.; Zimmerman, GA. & Prescott, SM. (2001). Altered expression of the mRNA stability factor HuR promotes cyclooxygenase-2 expression in colon cancer cells. *J Clin Invest.*, 108,1657-1665.

Edwards, JG.; Faux, SP.; Plummer, SM.; Abrams, KR.; Walker, RA.; Waller, DA. & O'Byrne KJ. (2002), Cyclooxygenase-2 expression is a novel prognostic factor in malignant mesothelioma. *Clin Cancer Res*, 8,1857-1862

Foster, JM.; Gatalica, Z:; Lilleberg, S.; Haynatzki, G. & Loggie, BW. (2009). Novel and existing mutations in the tyrosine kinase domain of the epidermal growth factor receptor are predictors of optimal resectability in malignant peritoneal mesothelioma. *Ann Surg Oncol*, 16,152-158

Foster, JM.; Radhakrishna, U.; Govindarajan, V.; Carreau, JH.; Gatalica, Z.; Sharma, P.; Nath, SK. & Loggie, BW. (2010). Clinical implications of novel activating EGFR mutations in malignant peritoneal mesothelioma. *World J Surg Oncol*, 8,88

Garland, LL.; Rankin, C.; Gandara, DR.; Rivkin, SE.; Scott, KM.; Nagle, RB.; Klein-Szanto, AJ.; Testa, JR.; Altomare, DA. & Borden, EC. (2007). Phase II study of erlotinib in patients with malignant pleural mesothelioma: a Southwest Oncology Group Study. *J Clin Oncol*, 25,2406-2413.

Govindan, R.; Kratzke, RA.; Herndon, JE.; Niehans, GA.; Vollmer, R.; Watson, D.; Green, MR. & Kindler, HL. (2005). Cancer and Leukemia Group B (CALGB 30101). Gefitinib in patients with malignant mesothelioma: a phase II study by the Cancer and Leukemia Group B. *Clin Cancer Res*, 11,2300–2304.

Greenhough, A.; Smartt, HJ.; Moore, AE.; Roberts, HR.; Williams, AC.; Paraskeva, C. & Kaidi, A. (2009). The COX-2/PGE2 pathway: key roles in the hallmarks of cancer and adaptation to the tumour microenvironment. Carcinogenesis, 30,377-386.

Gutkind,JS. (1998). The pathways connecting G protein-coupled receptors to the nucleus through divergent mitogen-activated protein kinase cascades. *J Biol Chem.*, 273, 1839–1842

Harris RE. Cyclooxygenase-2 (cox-2) and the inflammogenesis of cancer. Subcell Biochem. 2007;42:93-126. Review

Herbst, RS. (2004). Review of epidermal growth factor receptor biology. *Int. J. Radiat. Oncol. Biol. Phys.*, 59,21–26

Jänne, PA.; Taffaro, ML.; Salgia, R. & Johnson, BE (2002). Inhibition of epidermal growth factor receptor signaling in malignant pleural mesothelioma. *Cancer Res*, 62,5242-5247

Kamp, DW. & Weitzman, SA. (1999) The molecular basis of asbestos induced lung injury. *Thorax*, 54,638-652.

Kotani, M.; Tanaka, I.; Ogawa, Y.; Usui, T.; Mori, K.; Ichikawa, A.; Narumiya, S.; Yoshimi, T.; & Nakao, K. (1995) Molecular cloning and expression of multiple isoforms of human prostaglandin E receptor EP3 subtype generated by alternative messenger RNA splicing: multiple second messenger systems and tissue-specific distributions. *Mol Pharmacol* 48,869–879.

Kothmaier, H.; Quehenberger, F.; Halbwedl, I.; Morbini, P.; Demirag, F.; Zeren, H.; Comin, CE.; Murer, B.; Cagle, PT.; Attanoos, R.; Gibbs, AR.; Galateau-Salle, F.; Popper HH. (2008) EGFR and PDGFR differentially promote growth in malignant epithelioid mesothelioma of short and long term survivors. *Thorax* 63:345-351.

Krysan, K.; Reckamp, KL.; Dalwadi, H, Sharma S, Rozengurt E, Dohadwala M, Dubinett SM. (2005). Prostaglandin E2 activates mitogen-activated protein kinase/Erk pathway signaling and cell proliferation in non-small cell lung cancer cells in an epidermal growth factor receptor-independent manner. *Cancer Res*, 65,14,6275-6281.

Lippman, SM.; Gibson, N.; Subbaramaiah, K. & Dannenberg, AJ. (2005). Combined targeting of the epidermal growth factor receptor and cyclooxygenase-2 pathways. *Clin Cancer Res*. 11,17,6097-6099

Mineo, TC.; Ambrogi, V.; Cufari, ME. & Pompeo E. (2010). May cyclooxygenase-2 (COX-2), p21 and p27 expression affect prognosis and therapeutic strategy of patients with malignant pleura mesothelioma? *Eur J Cardiothorac Surg*., 38,3,245-52

Mossman, BT. & Churg, A. (1998). Mechanisms in the pathogenesis of asbestosis and silicosis. *Am J Respir Crit Care Med*., 157,1666-80.

Mossman, BT.; Kamp, DW. & Weitzman, SA. (1996). Mechanisms of carcinogenesis and clinical features of asbestos-associated cancers. *Cancer Invest*., 14,466-480.

Narumiya, S.; Sugimoto, Y. & Ushikubi, F. (1999). Prostanoid receptors: structures, properties, and functions. *Physiol Rev* 79,1193–1226

Neragi-Miandoab, S.; Richards, WG. & Sugarbaker, DJ. (2008). Morbidity, mortality, mean survival, and the impact of histology on survival after pleurectomy in 64 patients with malignant pleural mesothelioma. *Int J Surg* , 6,293–297

Nicholson, RI.; Gee, JMW. & Harper, ME. (2001) EGFR and cancer prognosis. *Eur J Cancer*., 37,S9–S15

Oda, K.; Matsuoka, Y.; Funahashi, A. & Kitano, H. (2005). A comprehensive pathway map of epidermal growth factor receptor signaling. *Mol. Syst. Biol*., 1,1.

O'Kane, SL.; Eagle, GL.; Greenman, J.; Lind, MJ. & Cawkwell, L. (2010). COX-2 specific inhibitors enhance the cytotoxic effects of pemetrexed in mesothelioma cell lines. *Lung Cancer*, 67,2,160-165.

Okuda, K.; Sasaki, H.; Kawano, O.; Yukiue, H.; Yokoyama, T.; Yano, M. & Fujii, Y. (2008). Epidermal growth factor receptor gene mutation, amplification and protein expression in malignant pleural mesothelioma. *J Cancer Res Clin Oncol*., 134,1105–1111

Orengo, AM.; Spoletini, L.; Procopio, A.; Favoni, RE.; De Cupis, A.; Ardizzoni, A.; Castagneto, B.; Ribotta, M.; Betta, PG.; Ferrini, S. & Mutti, L (1999). Establishment of four new mesothelioma cell lines: characterization by ultrastructural and immunophenotypic analysis *Eur Respir J* , 13,527-534

Ou, WB.; Hubert, C.; Corson, JM.; Bueno, R.; Flynn, DL.; Sugarbaker, DJ. & Fletcher JA. (2011). Targeted inhibition of multiple receptor tyrosine kinases in mesothelioma. *Neoplasia*, 13,1,12-22.

Pai, R.; Soreghan, B.; Szabo, IL.; Pavelka, M.; Baatar, D. & Tarnavski, AJ. (2002) Prostaglandin E2 transactivates EGF receptor: a novel mechanism for promoting colon cancer growth and gastrointestinal hypertrophy. *Na. Med* 8, 289–293

Pelucchi, C.; Malvezzi, M.; La Vecchia, C.; Levi F.; Decarli, A.& Negri, E. (2004).The Mesothelioma epidemic in Western Europe: an update. *Br J Cancer, 90,1022-1024.*

Pache, JC.; Janssen, YM.; Walsh, ES.; Quinlan, TR.; Zanella, CL.; Low, RB.; Taatjes, DJ. & Mossman, BT. (1998) Increased epidermal growth factor-receptor protein in a human mesothelial cell line in response to long asbestos fibers. *Am J Pathol* , 152,333–340.

Patrone, C.; Cassel, TN.; Pettersson, K.; Piao, YS.; Cheng, G.; Ciana, P.; Maggi, A.; Warner, M.; Gustafsson, JA. & Nord, M. (2003). Regulation of postnatal lung development and homeostasis by estrogen receptor beta. *Mol Cell Biol,* 23,8542–8552.

Peto, J.; Decarli, A.; La Vecchia, C.; Levi, F. & Negri E.(1999). The European mesothelioma epidemic. Br J Cancer. 79,666-672.

Pietras, RJ.; Marquez, DC.; Chen, HW.; Tsai, E.; Weinberg, O. & Fishbein, M. (2005). Estrogen and growth factor receptor interactions in human breast and non-small cell lung cancer cells. *Steroids*, 70,372–381.

Pinton, G.; Brunelli, E.; Murer, B.; Puntoni, R.; Puntoni, M.; Fennell, DA.; Gaudino, G.;
Mutti, L. & Moro, L. (2009). Estrogen receptor-beta affects the prognosis of human malignant mesothelioma *Cancer Res.*, 69,4598-4604

Prescott, SM. & Fitzpatrick, FA. (2000). Cyclooxygenase and carcinogenesis. *Biochim Biophys Acta,* 1470,2,M69-78.

Ramael, M.; Segers, K.; Buysse, C.; Van den Bossche, J. & Van Marck, E. (1991) .Immunohistochemical distribution patterns of epidermal growth factor receptor in malignant mesothelioma and non-neoplastic mesothelium. *Virchows Arch A Pathol Anat Histopathol.*, 419,171–175.

Reed, MJ.; Coldham, NG.; Patel, SR.; Ghilchik, MW. & James, VH. (1992). Interleukin-1 and interleukin-6 in breast cyst fluid: their role in regulating aromatase activity in breast cancer cells. *J Endocrinol.*, 132,R5-R8

Rena, O.; Boldorini, LR.; Gaudino, E. & Casadio, C. (2011). Epidermal growth factor receptor overexpression in malignant pleural mesothelioma: Prognostic correlations. *J Surg Oncol.*, Mar 21

Robinson, BW. & Lake, RA. (2005). Advances in malignant mesothelioma. *N Engl J Med.* ,353,1591-1603.

Sales, KJ.; Maudsley, S. & Jabbour, NH. (2005) Elevated Prostaglandin EP2 receptor in endometrial adenocarcinoma cells promotes vascular endothelial growth factor expression via cyclic 3_,5_-adenosin monophosphate-mediated transactivation of the epidermal growth factor receptor and extracellular signal-regulated kinase1/2 signaling pathways. *Mol. Endocrinol.*18, 1533–1545.

Scapoli, L.; Ramos-Nino, ME.; Martinelli, M.; Mossman, BT. (2004) Src-dependent ERK5 and Src/EGFR-dependent ERK1/2 activation is required for cell proliferation by asbestos. *Oncogene*,23:805-813.

Shukla, A.; Barrett, TF.; Macpherson, MB.; Hillegass, JM.; Fukagawa, NK.; Swain, WA.; O'Byrne,KJ.; Testa, JR.; Pass, HI.; Faux, SP. & Mossman BT. (2011). An ERK2 Survival Pathway Mediates Resistance of Human Mesothelioma Cells to Asbestos-Induced Injury. Am J *Respir Cell Mol Biol.*, Mar 31

Simoncini, T. & Genazzani, AR. (2003). Non-genomic actions of sex steroid hormones, *Eur J Endocrinol* 148,281–292.

Simoncini, T., Mannella, P., Fornari, L., Caruso, A.; Varone, G. & Genazzani, AR. (2004) .Genomic and non-genomic effects of estrogens on endothelial cells, *Steroids* 69,537–542

Stabile, LP.; Davis, AL.; Gubish, CT.; Hopkins, TM.; Luketich, JD.; Christie, N.; Finkelstein, S. & Siegfried, JM. (2002). Human non-small cell lung tumors and cells derived from normal lung express both estrogen receptor α and β and show biological responses to estrogen. *Cancer Res*, 62,2141–2150.

Stoppoloni, D.; Canino, C.; Cardillo, I.; Verdina, A.; Baldi, A.; Sacchi, A. & Galati, R. (2010). Synergistic effect of gefitinib and rofecoxib in mesothelioma cells. *Mol Cancer*, 9,27.

Stoppoloni, D.; Cardillo, I.; Verdina, A.; Vincenzi, B.; Menegozzo, S.; Santini, M.; Sacchi, A.; Baldi, A. & Galati, R. (2008). Expression of the embryonic lethal abnormal vision-like protein HuR in human mesothelioma: association with cyclooxygenase-2 and prognosis. *Cancer*, 113,2761-2769

Stoppoloni, D.; Salvatori, L.; Biroccio, A.; D'Angelo, C.; Muti, P.; Verdina, A.; Sacchi, A.; Vincenzi, B.; Baldi, A. & Galati R. (2011). Aromatase inhibitor exemestane has antiproliferative effects on human mesothelioma cells. *J Thorac Oncol*. 6,583-91

Travis, WD.; Colby, TV. & Corrin, B. (1999). Histological Typing of Lung and Pleural Tumours 3rd edn. Springer: Berlin.

Trupiano, JK.; Geisinger, KR., Willingham, MC.; Manders, P.; Zbieranski, N.; Case, D. & Levine, EA. (2004). Diffuse malignant mesothelioma of the peritoneum and pleura, analysis of markers. *Mod Pathol*. 17,476-481.

Vane, JR.; Mitchell, JA.; Appleton, I.; Tomlinson, A.; Bishop-Bailey, D.; Croxtall, J. &
Willoughby, DA. (1994). Inducible isoforms of cyclooxygenase and nitric-oxide synthase in inflammation. *Proc Natl Acad Sci USA*,91,2046-2050.

Veltman, JD.; Lambers, ME.; van Nimwegen, M.; Hendriks, RW.; Hoogsteden, HC.; Aerts, JG. & Hegmans, JP. (2010). COX-2 inhibition improves immunotherapy and is associated with decreased numbers of myeloid-derived suppressor cells in mesothelioma. Celecoxib influences MDSC function. *BMC Cancer*, 10,464.

Zahner, G., Wolf, G., Ayoub, M., Reinking, R., Panzer, U., Shankland, SJ. & Stahl RAK. (2002). Cyclooxygenase-2 overexpression inhibits platelet-derived growth factor-induced mesangial cell proliferation through induction of the tumor suppressor gene p53 and the cyclin-dependent kinase inhibitors p21waf-1/cip-1 and p27kip-1. *J Biol Chem*, 277,9763-9771

Zanella, CL., Posada, J.; Tritton, TR. & Mossman BT. (1996). Asbestos causes stimulation of the extracellular signal–regulated kinase 1 mitogen–activated protein kinase cascade after phosphorylation of the epidermal growth factor receptor. *Cancer Res*, 56,5334-5338.

Zhao, Y.; Agarwal, VR.; Mendelson, CR. & Simpson, ER. (1996). Estrogen biosynthesis proximal to a breast tumour is stimulated by PGE2 via cyclic AMP leading to activation of promoter II of the CYP19A1 (aromatase) gene. *Endocrinology*, 137,5739- 5742

Chapter 5

Neoadjuvant Chemotherapy in Malignant Pleural Mesothelioma

Giulia Pasello and Adolfo Favaretto

Additional information is available at the end of the chapter

http://dx.doi.org/10.5772/47880

1. Introduction

Malignant pleural mesothelioma (MPM) is a rare and aggressive tumour with a poor prognosis, directly related to chronic inhalation of asbestos fibres. Despite the extraction, import and marketing of the mineral were banned in most of the industrialized nations, the epidemiologic data foresee a sharp rise of MPM incidence and mortality in the next fifteen years because of the long lag time (even 40 years) from exposure to clinical evidence (Marinaccio et al., 2007).

Malignant mesothelioma is usually diagnosed in the advanced stages and single-modality treatment generally did not achieve higher results than supportive care. MPM shows high refractoriety to systemic treatment, and the response rate in previous series was about 10%-20% with anthracyclines, antimetabolites, or single agents platinum analogs.

Doublet chemotherapy showed similar results, even though some combinations yielded higher response rates than single agents. Responses are of short duration and complete responses are rarely observed. Currently available chemotherapy regimens achieved a response rate of 30-40% with rare complete responses, a median progression free and overall survival of approximately 6 and 12 months respectively (van Meerbeeck et al., 2005; Vogelzang et al., 2003).

With regard to local treatments, radiotherapy to the entire hemithorax may cause life-threatening pulmonary toxicity when the lung is not removed.

Extrapleural pneumonectomy (EPP), a surgical procedure introduced in the seventies which implies en bloc resection of the parietal pleurae, lung, ipsilateral pericardium and hemidiaphragm, did not improve the incidence of local and distant recurrences and that was the reason for some centres to perform combined treatments.

Multimodality therapies adopting a combination of surgical resection and adjuvant treatments (chemotherapy, radiotherapy or both) seem to be a better therapeutic option in selected patients (Sugarbaker et al., 1999); the successful results with neoadjuvant chemotherapy in the management of stage III Non-Small Cell Lung Cancer (Rosell et al., 1994) paved the way to several groups for applying this strategy in malignant mesothelioma.

Despite the improvement in diagnosis and treatment, the optimal therapy for mesothelioma patients is highly controversial and the role of surgery and trimodality treatment is under debate. There is no consensus about the benefits of neoadjuvant chemotherapy and about the more effective chemotherapy regimen, despite several clinical trials in this setting were performed.

2. Rationale for neoadjuvant treatment in malignant pleural mesothelioma

Treatment failure after surgery of malignant mesothelioma occurs frequently; in the attempt of reducing the incidence of local recurrences after extrapleural pneumonectomy, a multimodality approach with surgery followed by adjuvant radiotherapy was explored.

Extrapleural pneumonectomy allows higher doses of radiotherapy to the whole hemithorax by avoiding pulmonary toxicity and the results of this approach is a significant reduction of loco-regional relapses (Rusch et al., 2001).

The issue of extrathoracic metastasis represent a major challenge in the management of the disease because of the impact on overall survival (Rice et al., 2007)

Once a chemotherapy regimen showes activity in malignant pleural mesothelioma, the subsequent step is the addition of such treatment to surgery and radiotherapy to improve the systemic control of the disease.

The success with surgical resection after neoadjuvant chemotherapy in stage IIIA non-small cell lung cancer (Rosell et al., 1994) has been the impetus for several groups to apply this strategy in malignant mesothelioma aiming at reducing the incidence of distant relapse after surgery.

2.1. Neoadjuvant chemotherapy in non-small cell lung cancer

Until the nineties, local treatments such as surgery or radiotherapy were used alone to treat stage IIIA non-small cell lung cancer (locally invasive primary tumors or tumors associated with involvement of ipsilateral mediastinal or subcarineal lymphnodes). Five-years survival of non-small cell lung cancer patients is highly affected by stage of disease and lymphnodes involvement, and new approaches to improve overall survival has been investigated. The administration of systemic therapy before local treatment is generally referred to as induction or neoadjuvant therapy, and aims to prevent systemic spread of disease, to fight back micrometastasis and to reduce tumor size.

In 1994, two randomized clinical trials compared the combination of preoperative chemotherapy and surgery to surgery alone (Rosell et al., 1994; Roth et al., 1994). Median survival time, in two trials respectively, were 26 and 64 months in patients treated with platinum-based chemotherapy followed by surgery compared to 8 and 11 months, respectively, in the group who underwent to surgery alone. The effectiveness of such approach was confirmed in a systematic review and meta-analysis where data from 7 randomized clinical trials were available; the authors reported a 18% relative reduction in the risk of death, a significant increase of overall survival and an absolute benefit of 6 % at five years with the use of induction chemotherapy (Burdett et al., 2006, 2007). Subsequently, Song W. and colleagues, published an updated metanalysis with data from 13 studies, included 6 new randomized clinical trials; they reported a significant benefit in terms of overall survival in non-small lung cancer patients treated with chemotherapy followed by surgery compared to surgery alone, and the results were confirmed in the subgroup analysis where only stage III NSCLC patients were evaluated (Song et al., 2010).

2.2. Path to neoadjuvant chemotherapy in malignant pleural mesothelioma

The addition of systemic treatment to surgery and radiotherapy aims at reducing metastatic disease, even though the optimal sequence of the three is still unclear.

A major experience in surgical management of malignant mesothelioma was conducted by Sugarbaker et al. who tested the efficacy of extrapleural pneumonectomy followed by adjuvant chemotherapy and radiotherapy in 183 patients.

Chemotherapy regimen changed during study time window; doxorubicin and cyclophosphamide with or without cisplatin was administered in the first period, followed by carboplatin plus paclitaxel to later patients.

In their experience, patients with microscopic negative resection margins, epithelial histo-type and negative lymphnodes, had a better long-term survival (2 and 5 year survival: 68 and 46%, respectively; median 51 months) (Sugarbaker et al., 1999)

Patients with non-epithelial histology and extrapleural nodal involvement had worse survival and that underlines the need for a careful selection of patients undergoing a multimodality approach. A number of other studies were published with different regimens of adjuvant chemotherapy with a median overall survival of 13 to 23.9 months. Perioperative mortality in patients treated with adjuvant chemoradiotherapy ranged from 0 to 11% (Cao et al.,2010).

The difficult deliver of both postoperative chemotherapy and radiotherapy in most patients induced many groups to explore a trimodality approach based on preoperative chemotherapy, surgery and postoperative radiotherapy in the attempt of improving compliance.

Furthermore, as well as in non-small cell lung cancer, neoadjuvant chemotherapy could maximize cytoreduction and increase the proportion of patients able to complete the entire trimodality treatment.

3. Chemotherapy regimens in the neoadjuvant setting of malignant pleural mesothelioma

Recently the use of neoadjuvant chemotherapy has been reported in 7 prospective and 3 retrospective published studies, with median overall survival ranging from 23 to 33 months in patients who completed the trimodality treatement (Table 1, 2). Preliminary data are available from other clinical trials, and some studies are still ongoing.

Reference	Weder et al., 2004	Weder et al., 2007	Rea et al., 2007	Flores et al., 2006	Opitz et al., 2006
N° pts	19	61	21	21	63
Study type	Prospective	Prospective	Prospective	Prospective	Retrospective
CT	C-DDP 80 mg/m² d1 + G 1000 mg/m² d 1,8,15 every 28 days X 3	C-DDP 80 mg/m² d1 + G 1000 mg/m² d 1,8,15 every 28 days X 3	Cb AUC 5 d1 + G 1000 mg/m² d 1,8,15 every 28 days X 3-4	C-DDP 75 mg/m² d1 + G 1250 mg/m² d1,8 every 21 days X 3	Before 2003: C-DDP 80 mg/m² d1 + G 1000 mg/m² d 1,8,15 every 28 days X 3; After 2003: C-DDP 80 mg/m² d1 + P 500 mg/m² d1 every 21 days X 3
RR	32%	NR	33.3%	26%	32%
N° EPP	84%	74%	80.9%	42%	-
Peri-operative mortality rate	0%	2.2%	0%	0%	3.2%
RT	30 Gy in 2 Gy fractions + site specific boost to 60 Gy	50-60 Gy in 2 Gy fractions	45 Gy in 1.8 Gy fractions + boost 10-14 Gy in 2 Gy fractions	54 Gy in 1.8 fractions	30 Gy in 2 Gy fractions + boost 20 Gy or IMRT 45-55 Gy
TMT	68%	59%	71%	42%	-
OS (ITT)	23 months	19.8 months	25.5 months	19 months	NR
OS(EPP)	NR	CT + EPP: 23 months	27.5 months	CT + EPP + RT: 33.5 months	NR
PFS	CT + EPP: 16.5 months	CT + EPP: 13.5 months	CT + EPP: 16.3 months	NR	NR

Table 1. Summary of studies with gemcitabine plus a platinum compound as neoadjuvant chemotherapy regimen in malignant mesothelioma patients who underwent trimodality treatment. (EPP: extrapleural pneumonectomy; TMT: trimodality treatment; ITT: intention to treat; NR: not reported; IMRT: intensity modulated radiation therapy; OS: overall survival; PFS: progression free survival; RR: response rate; CDDP: cisplatin; G: gemcitabine; Cb: Carboplatin; P: pemetrexed; CT: chemotherapy; RT: radiotherapy)

Reference	Buduhan et al., 2009	de Perrot et al., 2009	Krug et al., 2009	Van Schil et al., 2010	Rea et al., 2011
N° pts	55	60	77	58	54
Study type	Retrospective	Retrospective	Prospective	Prospective	Prospective
CT	C-DDP/Cb +P; C-DDP + MTX+ Vb; C-DDP+ G; other	C-DDP +Vn; C-DDP+ P; C-DDP + R; C-DDP + G X 2-6	C-DDP + P X 3	C-DDP + P X 3	C-DDP + P X 3
RR	NR	NR	32.5%	43.9%	29.6%
N° EPP	84%	75%	70.1%	72.4%	83.3%
Peri-operative mortality rate	4.3%	6.7%	4%	6.5%	NR
RT	EBRT 30 Gy in 1.8-2 Gy fractions + boost 9-18 Gy or IMRT 50 Gy + boost 24 Gy	50 Gy in 2 Gy fractions + boost 10 Gy; or IMRT 54 Gy in 1.8 Gy fractions	54 Gy in 1.8 Gy fractions	54 Gy in 1.8 Gy fractions	54 Gy in 1.8 Gy fractions then emended to 50.4 Gy in 1.8 Gy fractions
TMT	69%	50%	52%	64.9%	40.7%
OS (ITT)	NR	14 months	16.8 months	18.4 months	15.5 months
OS (EPP)	CT + EPP: 24 months; TMT: 25 months	NR	CT+ EPP: 21.9 months: TMT: 29.1 months	TMT: 33 months	NR
PFS	NR	NR	ITT: 10.1 months; CT + EPP: 18.3 months	ITT: 13.9 months	ITT EFS: 6.9 months; ITT PFS: 8.6 months

Table 2. Summary of studies with pemetrexed plus a platinum compound as neoadjuvant chemotherapy regimen (EPP: extrapleural pneumonectomy; TMT: trimodality treatment; ITT: intention to treat; NR: not reported; NA: not available; EBRT: external beam radiotherapy; IMRT: intensity modulated radiation therapy; EFS: event free survival; OS: overall survival; PFS: progression free survival; RR: response rate; CDDP: cisplatin; G: gemcitabine; Cb: Carboplatin; P: pemetrexed; Vb: vinblastine; Vn: vinorelbine; R: raltitrexed; MTX: methotrexate; CT: chemotherapy; RT: radiotherapy)

When we analyze those results, we should consider the heterogeneity in terms of patient selection, treatment regimens, and methods for follow-up and overall survival analysis.

Over the years standard chemotherapy regimens for systemic treatment of malignant pleural mesothelioma has been changed.

On the basis of results in the metastatic disease, the association of carboplatin or cisplatin plus gemcitabine was considered as an effective treatment (Byrne et al.,1999; Nowak et al., 2002; Favaretto et al., 2003; Castagneto et al., 2005; Kalmadi et al., 2008).

In 2003 and 2005 two phase III trials were published which reported striking results when cisplatin was associated to pemetrexed and raltitrexed respectively, compared to cisplatin as single agent in mesothelioma patients who were not eligible for curative surgery. Those regimens achieved a response rate of 30-40%, a median progression free and overall survival of approximately 6 and 12 months respectively [(Van Meerbeeck et al., 2005; Vogelzang et al., 2003) .

After the two studies, a combination of cisplatin and an antifolate has become the golden standard in the first line treatment of malignant pleural mesothelioma patients not suitable for surgery and, subsequently, also in neoadjuvant setting.

3.1. Doublet chemotherapy with gemcitabine combined to a platinum compound

Since the end of the nineties, several groups analyzed the effectiveness and toxicity of gemcitabine combined to carboplatin or cisplatin in advanced mesothelioma patients (Byrne et al.,1999; Nowak et al., 2002; Favaretto et al., 2003; Castagneto et al., 2005; Kalmadi et al., 2008).

Those phase II trials showed a response rate ranging from 12% to 47%, an overall survival from 10 to 16 months, and a progression free survival from 6 to 10 months.

In the wake of the results by Byrne and colleagues in metastatic disease, in 2004 a Swiss group conducted a pilot study investigating neoadjuvant chemotherapy with cisplatin and gemcitabine followed by extrapleural pneumonectomy with or without adjuvant radiotherapy in 19 malignant pleural mesothelioma patients with resectable disease (Weder et al., 2004). Induction chemotherapy consisted of three cycles of cisplatin 80 mg/m^2 on day 1 *plus* gemcitabine 1000 mg/m^2 on day 1, 8, 15 every four weeks.

Extrapleural pneumonectomy was planned in all patients , while the total dose and fractionation of radiotherapy was decided according to resection margins and the target volume (hemitoracic three-dimensional conformal radiotherapy 30 to 60 Gy). 13 (68%) patients completed the entire trimodality treatment.

Response rate to neoadjuvant chemotherapy was 32%; median overall survival in the intention-to-treat population was 23 months and disease free survival in patients who received preoperative chemotherapy and extrapleural pneumonectomy was 16.5 months.

The authors observed a higher compliance to neoadjuvant compared to the adjuvant chemotherapy adopted in a previous study; in fact, the three cycles of chemotherapy were administered successfully in 95% of the patients. The preoperative systemic approach did not increase perioperative mortality rate, and the morbidity rate was in line with previous experience.

The good toxicity profile of chemotherapy regimen and the efficacy and activity results, higher than with other trimodality approaches, suggested further investigation of such treatment in a Swiss multicenter study (Weder et al., 2007).

The study investigated the feasibility of three cycles of cisplatin *plus* gemcitabine at the same doses previously adopted, followed by extrapleural pneumonectomy and adjuvant radiotherapy up to 60 Grey to the involved hemithorax, in 61 patients.

Quality of life assessment was one of the endpoints of the study.

Chemotherapy was administered to 95% of the patients, while the resection rate was 74%. Complete resection (R0-R1) was achieved in 37 (61%) of the 45 patients who underwent EPP.

Trimodality treatment was completed by 36 (59%) patients, with an overall survival of 19.8 months in the intent-to-treat analysis and 23 months in patients who received both chemotherapy and surgery with or without adjuvant radiotherapy (Fig.1).

Median time to progression was 13.5 months, while no radiologic response rate was reported in the study. No significant worsening of quality of life was showed during the multimodality treatement. The postoperative mortality (2.2%) and the morbidity rate (35%) were acceptable and underline the need for experienced centre to follow such approach.

Considering the risk of increasing perioperative complications and postoperative mortality with the use of neoadjuvant chemotherapy, the administration of a chemotherapy regimen with lower toxicity seemed attractive.

Since 1996, our italian group tested the activity of carboplatin plus gemcitabine in a phase II study in 50 mesothelioma patients (Favaretto et al., 2003). We observed partial response in 26% of the patients, a median overall survival and progression free survival of about 16 and 10 months respectively, and an acceptable toxicity profile.

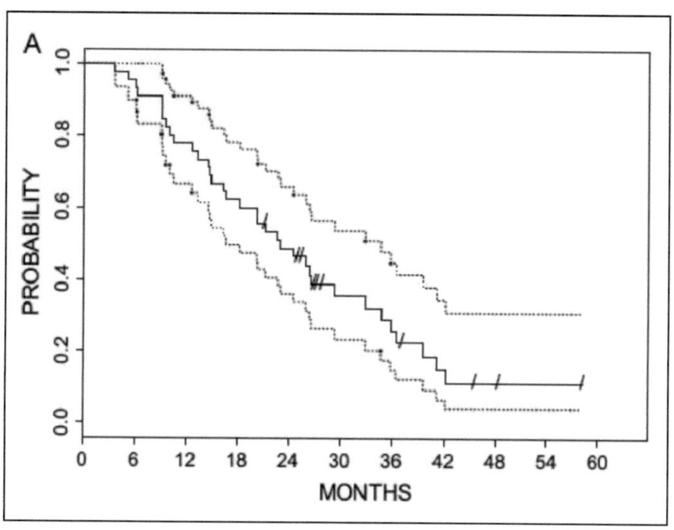

Figure 1. Overall survival in the intention-to-treat population .

Those results led us to evaluate the same chemotherapy combination in the neoadjuvant setting of a multimodality approach in 21 patients with resectable disease (Rea et al., 2007). Patients with stage I to III, epithelial or mixed mesothelioma underwent three to four cycles of chemotherapy with carboplatin [area under the concentration –time curve (AUC) 5] on day 1 and gemcitabine 1000 mg/m^2 on days 1,8,15 every four weeks. Patients with complete or partial response or stable disease underwent to extrapleural pneumonectomy within 4-6 weeks. Postoperative radiotherapy consisted of 45 Grey in 25 fractions to the hemitorax, with a boost dose of 10-14 Grey to high risk areas.

At the reassessment after induction chemotherapy, we observed 7 (33.3%) partial response and 14 (66.7%) stable disease.

The operability rate was about 81%, and 71% of the patients completed the trimodality protocol.

The median overall survival was 25.5 months in the intent-to-treat population, and 27.5 months in patients who received extrapleural pneumonectomy (Fig. 2). Median time to relapse was 16.3 months.

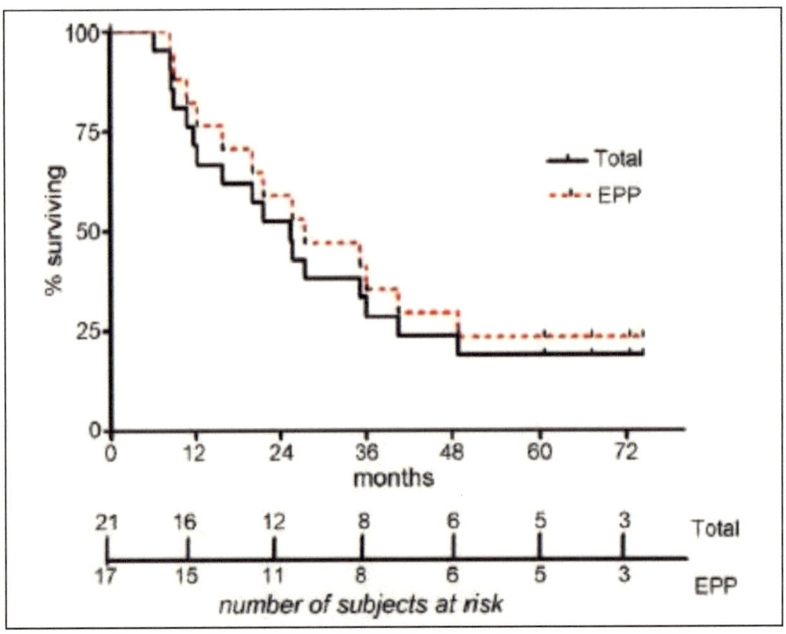

Figure 2. Overall survival in the intention to treat population and in patients who underwent extrapleural pneumonectomy for malignant pleural mesothelioma (Rea et al., 2007)

No intraoperative or perioperative morbidity was shown, while major complications were observed in 23.8% of the operated patients.

The absence of postoperative mortality characterizes another prospective study conducted at the Memorial Sloan-Kettering Cancer Center (Flores et al., 2006).

From 2002 to 2004, 21 patients with locally advanced mesothelioma (stage III-IV) were entered into a phase II trial designed to test the feasibility of induction chemotherapy with cisplatin and gemcitabine followed by extrapleural pneumonectomy and external beam hemithoracic radiotherapy (EBRT). Chemotherapy included 4 cycles of gemcitabine 1250 mg/m^2 on days 1,8 combined with cisplatin 75 mg/m^2 on day 1 every 21 days. Extrapleural pneumonectomy was performed within 3-5 weeks, in those patients who had resectable disease, followed by EBRT 54 Gy/30F starting 3-6 weeks after surgery. 19 patients started chemotherapy and 53% of them completed 4 cycles. Eight patients underwent EPP followed by EBRT, thus 42% of patients who completed the trimodality treatement.

Response to chemotherapy were: 26% partial response, 32% stable disease, 42% progressive disease.

Seven patients had grade 3 toxicity and one had grade 4 toxicity during chemotherapy, while only 2 (25%) grade 3 and no grade 4 surgical complications occurred. Median overall survival in the intent-to-treat population and in patients who completed also the surgical procedure and radiotherapy was 19 and 33.5 months respectively. The rationale of the trial was to test the multimodality approach in high-risk patients with advanced disease, to reduce the risk of systemic relapase and to improve the outcome of those patients.

The study was prematurely interrupted because of another prospective competitive trial ongoing at the Center.

Those prospective studies adopting gemcitabine as the third-generation agent associated to platinum in the neoadjuvant setting agree that systemic treatment before surgery did not increase mortality and morbidity rate, provided that trimodality approach was managed by an experienced multidisciplinary team.

A retrospective study on 63 mesothelioma patients published in 2006 by the Swiss group (Opitz et al., 2006) aimed at investigating the incidence of postoperative complications in the context of trimodality treatment.

Most of the patients (75%), who were included in the study before 2003, received three cycles of chemotherapy with cisplatin 80 mg/m^2 on day 1 *plus* gemcitabine 1000 mg/m^2 on day 1, 8, 15 every four weeks. Since 2003 the patients (25%) received induction chemotherapy based on three cycles of cisplatin 80 mg/m^2 *plus* pemetrexed 500 mg/m^2 on day 1 every three weeks.

Chemotherapy was followed by extrapleural pneumonectomy and radiotherapy (45 to 60 Grey to involved hemithorax including high risk areas).

Morbidity and mortality rate were 62% and 3.2 % respectively. The most frequent postoperative complication was empyema (15.8%), which was often associated to a longer duration of surgery. Other complications were chylothorax, patch failure, bleeding, herniation. Those complications were successfully managed by the surgical equipe, thanks to an increasing expertise during the years. Furthermore, the authors could predict and earlier treat those patients at higher risk of postoperative complications according to EORTC score, improving short-term outcome.

3.2. The advent of modern antifolate agents

Pemetrexed is an antifolate agent which inhibits three target enzymes involved in purine and pyrimidine synthesis: dihydrofolate reductase, thymidylate synthase and glycinamide ribonucleotide formyltransferase.

On the basis of encouraging results of phase I trials in malignant pleural mesothelioma and a phase II study in non-small cell lung cancer, Vogelzang and colleagues conducted a phase III trial of pemetrexed, an antifolate agent, plus cisplatin compared to cisplatin as a single agent in 456 mesothelioma patients who were not elegible for curative surgery.

The doublet regimen achieved a significant improvement in terms of overall survival (12.1 *versus* 9.3 months, $p= 0.02$), time to progression (5.7 *versus* 3.9 months, $p=0.001$) and response rate (41.3% *versus* 16.7%, $p< 0.0001$) compared to single agent chemotherapy (Vogelzang et al., 2003).

Two years later, data from another phase III trial were published, which showed a benefit in terms of overall (11.4 *versus* 8.8 months, $p= 0.048$) and progression free survival (5.3 *versus* 4.0 months, $p= 0.058$), and response rate (23.6% *versus* 13.6%, $p= 0.056$) among patients treated with cisplatin plus raltitrexed, a different thymidylate synthase inhibitor, compared to cisplatin alone (Van Meerbeeck et al., 2005).

As previously mentioned, the combination of ciplatin to an antifolate agent became the golden standard in the systemic treatment of advanced malignant pleural mesothelioma.

More recent neoadjuvant trials have investigated the outcomes of trimodality treatment with this new regimen (Buduhan et al., 2009; De Perrot et al., 2009; Krug et al., 2009; Rea et al., 2011; Van Schil et al., 2010).

3.2.1. *Retrospective studies*

Two retrospective studies published in 2009 analyzed the outcomes of mesothelioma patients treated with neoadjuvant chemotherapy before surgery and radiotherapy. Chemotherapy regimen consisted of platinum-based doublet combined to different drugs, even if during the study time it was standardized to cisplatin plus pemetrexed.

The study by the Swedish Medical Center Institute (Buduhan et al., 2009), reviewed a consecutive group of 46 mesothelioma patients who were eligible for trimodality treatment. Preoperative chemotherapy administerd to the initial cohort of 55 patients was based on a platinum compound plus pemetrexed (44%), cisplatin plus methotrexate plus vinblastine (41%), cisplatin plus gemcitabine (9%), other (5%). Mediastinoscopy was performed within 3-5 weeks after completion of chemotherapy in those patients eligible for surgery, and the finding of malignant nodes was an absolute contraindication to extrapleural pneumonectomy. However, 44% of the patients were node positive at resection.

Extrapleural pneumonectomy was feasible in 46 patients (84%), followed by adjuvant radiotherapy in 38 patients within 6-8 weeks from surgery.

During the study time frame, radiotherapy was administered according to two different modalities: conventional external beam radiotherapy (EBRT) to a median dose of 30 Gy in fractions of 1.8-2 Gy (63% of the patients) or intensity-modulated radiotherapy (IMRT) at the median dose of 50.4 Gy/28 F, with higher doses up to 60 Gy to the areas of residual disease (34% of the patients).

Trimodality treatment was completed by 69% of the initial cohort and median survival time for those patients was 25 months; nodal positivity and macroscopically positive margins were considered as predictors of worse survival.

Postoperative mortality rate was 4.3%; major comorbidities were present in 80% of the patients who underwent extrapleural pneumonectomy. Recurrent disease occurred in half of the patients in the ipsilateral hemithorax and it was more common among patients treated with EBRT compared to patients who received IMRT.

The main limitation of that study is the retrospective review of patients who started chemotherapy at different sites, so that it was not possible to determine which patients were selected for the trimodality treatment.

A mono-institutional experience was published during the same year (DePerrot et al., 2009), which retrospectively reviewed 60 cases of malignant pleural mesothelioma prospectively included in a trimodality protocol with induction chemotherapy, followed by extrapleural pneumonectomy and adjuvant high-dose hemithoracic radiation up to at least 50 Gy. Patients with sarcomatoid mesothelioma were excluded.

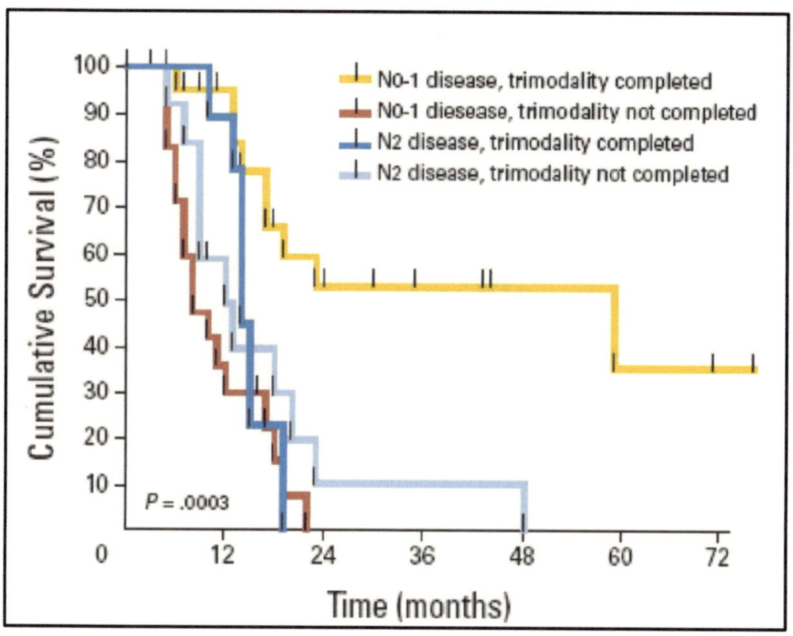

Figure 3. Survival according to mediastinal lymphonodes involvement and completion of the trimodality protocol, de Perrot et al., 2009

Induction chemotherapy consisted of cisplatin combined with one of the following agents: vinorelbine (43%), pemetrexed (40%), raltitrexed (10%), gemcitabine (7%) for 2 to 6 cycles. Grade 3 (leucopenia) and 4 (pulmonary embolism) toxicity was described in 1(2%) and 3(5%) patients respectively.

45 patients (75%) underwent extrapleural pneumonectomy, without significant difference between the induction regimens, while only half of the study population completed the trimodality treatment.

Complete resection was shown in 91% of the patients undergoing surgery. The perioperative mortality rate was 6.7%.

Median overall survival in the intention-to-treat population was 14 months; chemotherapy regimen had no impact on overall survival, which was significantly better in patients without mediastinal node involvement who completed the trimodality treatment (59 months compared to 8 months in patients without node involvement but who did not complete the trimodality protocol). N2 involvement was a negative prognostic factor, without any difference between patients who completed or not the protocol. Nodal status showed a significant impact also on disease free survival (Fig.3).

Therefore, the conclusion of the study was to exclude patients with N2 disease from a trimodality protocol.

As well as in the study by Buduhan, also the retrospective analysis by de Perrot was limited by the administration of different chemotherapy regimens during the study time frame.

After the publication by Vogelzang, several prospective clinical trials which evaluated cisplatin plus pemetrexed as standard induction chemotherapy were designed.

3.2.2. Prospective trials

On the basis of the favourable results by Vogelzang, a multicenter phase II trial from the Memorial Sloan-Kettering Cancer Center group chose pemetrexed and cisplatin as induction chemotherapy regimen before extrapleural pneumonectomy and adjuvant radiotherapy, to assess the feasibility of such trimodality protocol (Krug et al., 2009).

A cohort of 77 patients was included in the protocol, but only 64 (83.1%) completed four cycles of neoadjuvant chemotherapy with pemetrexed 500 mg/m^2 plus cisplatin 75 mg/m^2 on day 1 every three weeks. Extrapleural pneumonectomy was completed in 70.1% of the study population, while the trimodality protocol was completed by 40 (52%) patients.

Radiological response to induction chemotherapy was: 1 (1.3%) complete response, 24 (31.2%) partial response, 36 (46.8%) stable disease, 5 (6.5%) progressive disease and 11 (14.3%) patients with unknown or unavailable response.Three (5.3%) pathological complete response were reported. Grade 3-4 haematological toxicity was observed in 7.8% of the patients. The postoperative mortality was 4% and the rate of postoperative complication was in line with the studies we reported previously.

Median survival and progression free survival in the intent-to-treat population were 16.8 and 10.1 months respectively (Fig.4). Overall survival was higher in those patients who completed extrapleural pneumonectomy (21.9 months) and radiotherapy (29.1 months). Furthermore, radiologic response to induction chemotherapy was demonstrated as a significant prognostic factor: patients with complete or partial response had a median overall survival of 26 months compared to 13.9 months in patients with stable and progressive disease. Recurrences occurred in 40.4% of the patients who underwent extrapleural pneumonectomy, with a median time to relapse of 18.3 months.

The study by Krug and colleagues was the largest prospective trial of trimodality treatment, and shows toxicity and efficacy data in line with previous studies. The authors emphasized the importance of patients selection and team experience in the management of early stage malignant pleural mesothelioma.

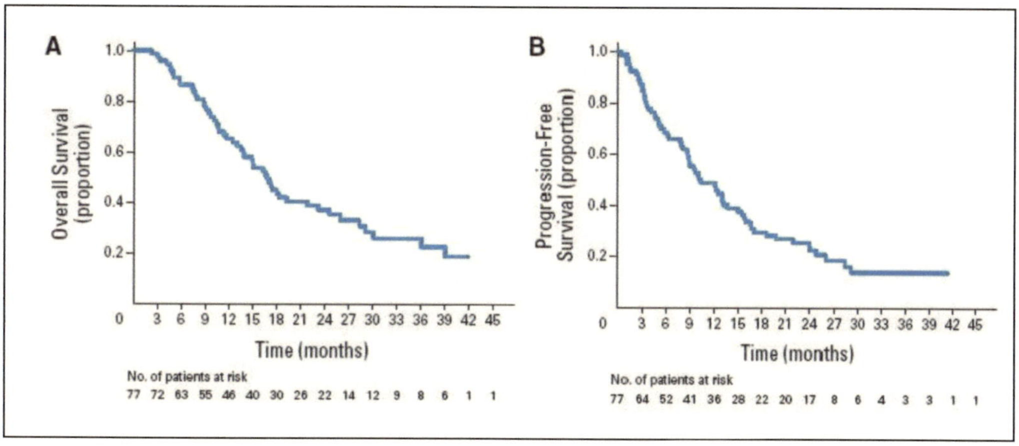

Figure 4. Overall survival (A) and progression free survival (B) in the intention to treat population of the study by Krug et al., 2009

The combination of cisplatin and pemetrexed was the induction regimen adopted from 2005 to 2007 in the multicenter study by European Organization for Research and Treatment of Cancer (EORTC) (Van Schil et al., 2010).

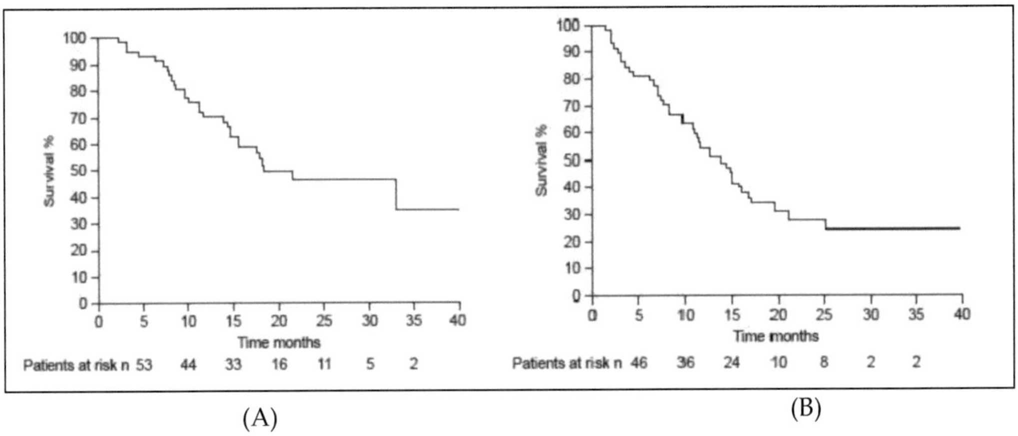

Figure 5. Overall survival and progression free survival (B) in the study population by Van Schil et al., 2010)

The primary endpoint of the study was to evaluate the "success of treatment" of a trimodality protocol based on induction chemotherapy with three cycles of cisplatin 75 mg/m^2 and pemetrexed 500 mg/m^2 every three weeks followed by extrapleural pneumonectomy within 3-8 weeks after the last chemotherapy cycle and adjuvant hemithoracic radiotherapy (54 Gy/30 F).

Success of treatment was defined as the completion of the trimodality protocol within the defined time frames and a survival of 90 days without progression or grade 3-4 toxicity. Overall survival, progression free survival and toxicity were secondary endpoints.

58 patients were included in the study, 57 of them started chemotherapy and 55 (94%) completed three cycles of chemotherapy. Extrapleural pneumonectomy was performed in 72.4%of the eligible patients, while 63.8% received also radiotherapy and completed the trimodality protocol.

Grade 3-4 toxicity after chemotherapy was observed in 27.7% of the patients, and persisted in 5.7% of the study population 90 days after the end of the protocol.

Radiological response at the end of induction chemotherapy was: complete in 24.6%, partial in 19.3%, stable in 42.1%, progressive in 8.8% and not assessable in 5.3% of the patients. After surgery, postoperative complications were described in 82.6% of the patients, while postoperative mortality rate was 6.5%. The primary endpoint was reached in 42.1% of the patients, that was lower than the 60% success rate needed to further investigate the trimodality treatment.

Median overall survival in the intention-to-treat population and in patients who completed the trimodality protocol was 18.4 and 33 months respectively; progression free survival for 57 eligible patients was 13.9 months (Fig.5).

The predefined criteria of successful treatment were set looser, a higher number of patients reached the primary endpoint. The study remarked that trimodality treatment should be considered in centers with high levels of expertise and in the context of prospective clinical trials for selected early stage malignant mesothelioma patients.

A recent prospective phase II study presented at the latest ASCO (American Society of Clinical Oncology) meeting by our group evaluated neoadjuvant chemotherapy with pemetrexed plus cisplatin followed by extrapleural pneumonectomy (Rea et al., 2011) and hemithoracic radiation in 54 mesothelioma patients.

Chemotherapy was administered every three weeks for three cycles, at the following doses: cisplatin 75 mg/m^2 and pemetrexed 500 mg/m^2. Surgery was performed within 3 weeks after chemotherapy; radiotherapy maximum dose was changed during the study from 54 Gy to 50.4 Gy, and the local radiation was planned within 4-12 weeks after extrapleural pneumonectomy. Chemotherapy was completed in 96%of the study population, while the trimodality treatment was completed in 22 (40.7%) patients.

Out of 54 patients, 16 (29.6%) showed partial response at the radiological assessment, 31 (57.4%) showed stable disease, 4 (7.4%) showed progressive disease.

Median event free survival was 6.9 months, median progression free survival: 8.6 months; median overall survival: 15.5 months; 67% of the patients experienced grade 3-4 toxicity.

In line with the previous studies in the same setting, the trimodality protocol presented in the study seemed feasible with manageable toxicity, provided that cardiopulmonary function is closely monitored.

3.3. The MARS trial

What is the chance of extrapleural pneumonectomy in the management of malignant pleural mesothelioma? This was the big question from which the Mesothelioma And Radical Surgery (MARS) trial rose in 2005 (Treasure et al.,2006, 2009, 2011) (Fig. 6).

The aim of the study was to put an end to the debate between believers and doubters about that surgical procedure, through a randomization between induction chemotherapy followed by extrapleural pneumonectomy and induction chemotherapy without EPP.

Initially, to assess the patients' compliance and the recruitment rate, a feasibility exploratory analysis was performed which randomized 50 patients in 1 year between the two treatment arms. The randomization seemed to be feasible in 45% of the patients included in the study, and a larger trial was published two years later, with the aim of evaluating the clinical outcome in randomly assigned patients.

The MARS study was a multicenter randomized controlled trial in 12 United Kingdom hospitals, with a two-stage consent process, before registration and before randomization (Fig.6).

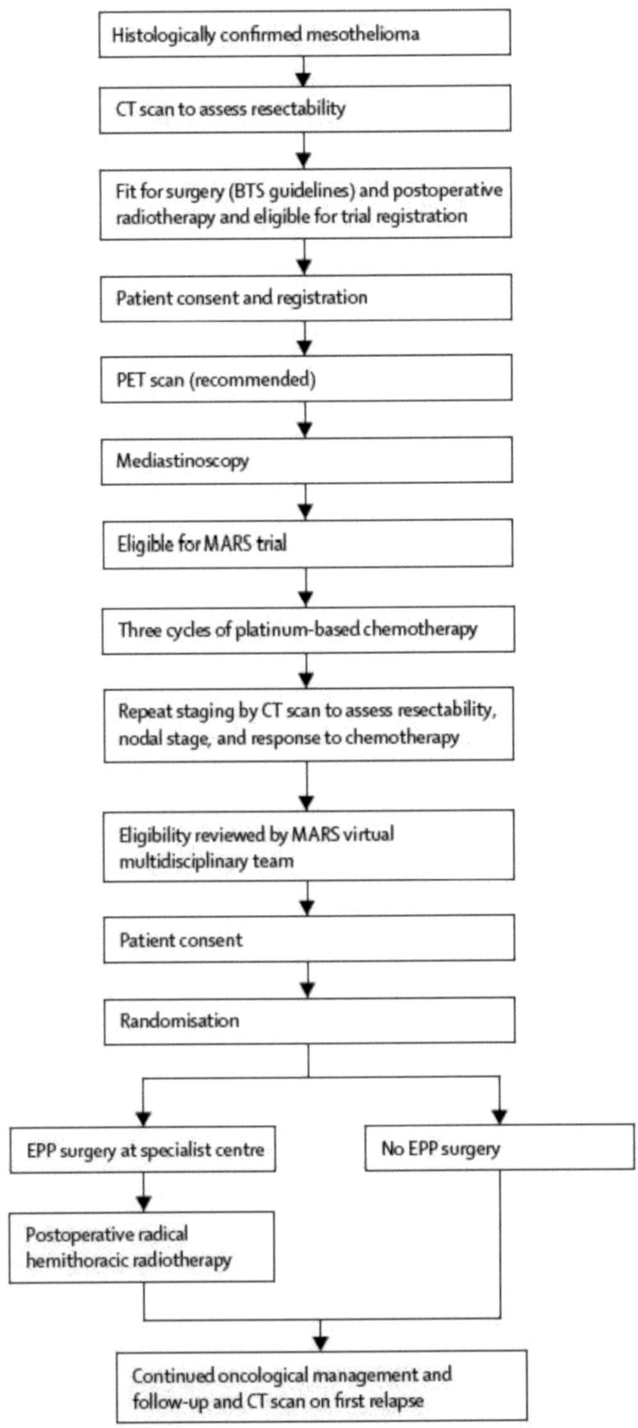

Figure 6. Study design of the Mesothelioma And Radical Surgery (MARS) trial.

After the first informed consent and registration, 112 patients underwent mediastinoscopy and PET, then 94 received at least one cycle of chemotherapy; in particular 83 (74%) of them received three cycles of platinum-based chemotherapy. The most common chemotherapy regimen adopted was cisplatin and gemcitabine (40%), followed by cisplatin and pemetrexed (26%), cisplatin and mitomycin and vinblastine (21%). At the end of chemotherapy patients underwent CT scan and they were re-evaluated for the eligibility to extrapleural pneumonectomy.

A second informed consent was provided to 50 patients before randomization. The proportion of patients who accepted to enter the registration phase was carefully documented.

Patients in the control arm were eligible for any oncological treatment, which included chemotherapy, radiotherapy, every surgical procedure but EPP, full supportive care.

24 patients were assigned to extrapleural pneumonectomy, 26 to no EPP. Among patients in the first group, 16 (67%) completed extrapleural pneumonectomy; perioperative deaths occurred in 15.8% of the patients and perioperative complications in 69% of the patients. Half of the patients who underwent extrapleural pneumonectomy received radiotherapy.

As far as the second group is concerned, further oncological treatment was administered to 32% of them; in particular, three patients received extrapleural pneumonectomy outside the trial. Among the 30 deaths within the first 24.7 months from randomization, 4 were perioperative events: 3 in the EPP arm, and 1 in the no EPP arm which occurred in a patient who underwent EPP outside the clinical trial.

Median survival from randomization was 14.4 months in patients addressed to EPP and 19.5 months in patients who did not undergo extrapleural pneumonectomy (p=0.016, after adjustment for prognostic factors). Median recurrence free survival in EPP group was 7.6 months; median progression free survival in no EPP group was 9.0 months.

Median quality of life seemed better in those patients who did not undergo extrapleural pneumonectomy; the lowest scores in EPP group were observed shortly after surgery.

The MARS trial was the first study which randomized between extrapleural pneumonectomy and no extrapleural pneumonectomy in the management of malignant pleural mesothelioma. The study population was small but the conclusion of the trial raised the issue of a less invasive approach as suitable treatment of malignant pleural mesothelioma. Those results are supported by previous data from the surgical group of Flores where extrapleural pneumonectomy was compared to pleurectomy/decortication in a multi-institutional trial where 663 patients consecutively underwent one of the two surgical procedures. The mortality rate was higher in patients treated with extrapleural pneumonectomy (7%) compared to patients who underwent pleurectomy/decortication (4%) (Flores et al., 2008)..

Overall survival was longer in those patients who were treated with pleurectomy/decortication; however gender, stage, histotype were significant factors which impacted the patients' outcome.

In the future, a randomized study to evaluate the outcome of patients treated with pleurectomy/decortication is needed.

4. Risks and benefits of neoadjuvant chemotherapy of malignant pleural mesothelioma

Platinum-based chemotherapy plus gemcitabine or pemetrexed for 3 to 4 cycles followed by surgery and postoperative high-dose radiotherapy showed the best results in terms of overall and progression free survival. However, patients were selected without a control group, and a randomized controlled trial to define the best treatment is still lacking.

Multimodality treatment is long. For the remarkable physical and psychological distress at the end of this invasive approach it is important to look for a strong evidence of the benefits.

The MARS trial tried to answer the question about the benefits of extrapleural pneumonectomy in the context of trimodality treatment. The results were controversial, so the debate inside the scientific community is still open.

Some thoracic surgeons and clinicians believe there is sufficient evidence to support the use of extrapleural pneumonectomy in selected patients; on the other side, the "doubters" underline the scientific bias inside the patients' selection: the improvement in overall survival with EPP might be the result of the exclusion of patients not suitable for surgery, therefore with unfavourable features.

The MARS study was the only randomized trial which compared EPP to no EPP, showing no benefit for mesothelioma patients who underwent such surgical procedure.

The optimal treatment for malignant pleural mesothelioma is still a matter of debate not only as far as the surgery is concerned.

In the context of a multimodality treatment, chemotherapy was administered as adjuvant treatment after surgery for many years, while the administration of chemotherapy in the induction phase was recently introduced in the clinical practice.

As already mentioned, the potential benefits of preoperative chemotherapy are the early eradication of the circulating metastases and the shrinkage of tumor size; the first could reduce the rate of distant recurrences and the second could make the surgery possible for inoperable tumors or easier for operable but extensive disease. Furthermore, the difficult delivery of both radiotherapy and chemotherapy after surgery was another reason to administer chemotherapy as the first step of the trimodality protocol aiming at a better tolerance of the side effects.

On the other side the delay of the surgical procedure is a disadvantage of neoadjuvant chemotherapy, especially when chemotherapy is not effective

Some authors reported the impairment of cardiorespiratory function as another detrimental effect of induction chemotherapy and showed an increased risk of perioperative morbidity and mortality.

4.1. Effects of neoadjuvant chemotherapy on the risk of perioperative morbidity and mortality

Many chemotherapeutic agents can cause lung and heart damage even if the type of the injury and its pathogenesis is unclear; however, the alveolo-capillary membrane seems to be the main target of chemotherapy.

Several evidences reported an increased mortality rate and risk of respiratory complications after induction chemotherapy in lung cancer, especially in those patients who received pneumonectomy.

In 2005, data from 74 mesothelioma patients who underwent EPP were analyzed to assess the incidence of perioperative complications (Stewart et al., 2005).

The authors identified three preoperative variables associated to perioperative complications.

Neoadjuvant chemotherapy with cisplatin doublet in combination with gemcitabine (9), pemetrexed (5) or vinorelbine (1) was administered in 20% of the study population, and it was associated to a higher risk of acute lung injury and symptomatic mediastinal shift. Long-standing operations were associated to increased risk of technical and gastrointestinal complications; finally, procedures on the right lung seemed to increase the risk of postoperative pneumonia and overall risk of perioperative mortality.

On the basis of previous results, our group conducted a prospective study to evaluate the effect of neoadjuvant chemotherapy on lung function and exercise capacity in 36 mesothelioma patients suitable for extrapleural pneumonectomy (Marulli et al., 2010).

Pulmonary function tests were performed twice: after the diagnostic video-assisted thoracoscopic surgery and before the first cycle of chemotherapy, and then four weeks after the last chemotherapy cycle. The tests comprised a spirometry with the measurement of slow and forced vital capacity (Vc and FVC), forced expiratory volume in the first second (FEV1), total lung capacity and diffusing capacity of the lung for carbon monoxide (DLCO); and an incremental exercise test using a cycle ergometer to assess the oxygen uptake (VO_2), CO_2 production (VCO_2) and minute ventilation (VE). Blood gas analysis was also performed.

Among the 36 patients included in the study, 52.8% received three cycles of induction chemotherapy with carboplatin (AUC 5) and pemetrexed (500 mg/m^2) on day 1 every three weeks; 47.2% received pemetrexed with cisplatin (75 mg/m^2) on day 1 every 21 days.

Radiologic assessment after chemotehrapy showed a 44.5% partial response, stable disease in 47.2% and progressive disease in 8.3%. Performance status after induction chemotherapy improved in 27.8%, was stable in 50% and worsened in 22.2% of the patients.

All the parameters estimated for the lung function and exercise tests improved after preoperative chemotherapy; in particular FEV1, oxygen pressure (PaO_2) at rest and at the peak of exercise and VO_2. A significant improvement of the lung volume indexes was observed in particular for those patients who achieved a partial response to induction chemotherapy; the results of the stratified analysis by response were explained by the cytoreductive effects of chemotherapy on the tumor mass, thus improving the lung expansion.

As already mentioned, chemotherapy could affect the lung function by decreasing the efficiency of alveolar-capillary membrane. In our study, gas exchange parameters were not impacted by induction chemotherapy, probably related to an improvement in alveolar volume. Preoperative chemotherapy seemed not to compromise the cardiopulmonary effectiveness to undergo EPP; such conclusion seems in line with the results of previous studies about trimodality treatment, which did not show increased perioperative mortality (table 1 and 2).

5. Potential benefits of a less aggressive approach in the management of malignant pleural mesothelioma: Which is the best chemotherapy regimen?

Trimodality treatment is one of the more invasive approaches in cancer management, and patients might suffer from perioperative complications due to the impaired clinical conditions after induction treatments.

Two surgical techniques are applied to the removal of malignant pleural mesothelioma: extrapleural pneumonectomy and pleurectomy/decortication.

Extrapleural pneumonectomy consists of en bloc resection of the pleura, lung, diaphragm, and pericardium, while pleurectomy/decortication removes the involved pleura and makes the underlying lung free to expand and fill the pleural cavity.

Despite previous studies did not show a significant rising in mortality and morbidity within trimodality protocols (Buduhan et al., 2009; De Perrot et al., 2009; Flores et al., 2006; Krug et al., 2009; Opitz et al., 2006; Rea et al., 2007, 2011; Van Schil et al., 2010, Weder et al., 2004, 2007) extrapleural pneumonectomy is still a controversial approach, especially in the light of the MARS trial results (Treasure et al., 2011).

The choice of extrapleural pneumonectomy (EPP) rather than pleurectomy/decortication (P/D) is not based on scientific evidences but on the surgeon decision.

In 2008, Flores and his group analyzed the outcome of the two surgical procedures in 663 malignant pleural mesothelioma patients (Flores et al., 2008). 60% of the study population received extrapleural pneumonectomy with a perioperative mortality of 7%. Perioperative mortality in the patients who received pleurectomy/decortication was 4%.

The decision to perform EPP rather than P/D was based on patients' clinical condition, intraoperative findings and tumor stage.

In the EPP group there was a higher proportion of patients who received a multimodality treatment, while in P/D group, elderly patients and early stage tumors were included.

Median overall survival and 5 –year survival in all the patients were 14 months and 12% respectively. Significant prognostic variables were stage, gender, asbestos exposure, histology, and multimodality treatment.

When overall survival was analyzed in the two subgroups, extrapleural pneumonectomy was associated to a worse prognosis, irrespective of stage and perioperative mortality (12 versus 16 months, $p<0.001$). The difference seemed less evident when survival data were analyzed in a multivariate analysis with other prognostic factors.

The main limitation of the study was the retrospective data analysis which did not allow any definitive conclusion about the outcome of the two surgical procedures.

In line with the results of the MARS study, a randomized trial which analyze the impact of pleurectomy/decortication on the overall survival of mesothelioma patients could define the role of lung-sparing surgery within a trimodality protocol.

As already mentioned, the role of chemotherapy in the multimodality management of malignant pleural mesothelioma aims at reducing distant recurrences.

So far, no randomized trial has compared different chemotherapy regimens in the induction phase of a trimodality protocol.

It is possible that the integration of less invasive treatments lead to a better outcome of mesothelioma patients.

Carboplatin is often preferred to cisplatin in the systemic treatment of cancer because it shows a lower incidence of neurotoxicity, nephrotoxicity, nausea and vomiting. When carboplatin substituted cisplatin in malignant pleural mesothelioma patients not eligible for surgery, it showed comparable results in terms of activity (Castagneto et al., 2008; Ceresoli et al., 2006; Favaretto et al., 2003).

Recently, our group retrospectively analyzed the feasibility of pemetrexed plus carboplatin or cisplatin as preoperative chemotherapy of malignant pleural mesothelioma (Pasello et al., 2011). 54 patients were consecutively included in a trimodality protocol based on preoperative chemotherapy followed by surgery and adjuvant radiotherapy; neoadjuvant chemotherapy was based on three cycles of pemetrexed (500 mg/m^2) plus carboplatin (AUC5) on day 1 every three weeks in 30 patients; 24 patients received pemetrexed (500 mg/m^2) plus cisplatin (75 mg/ m^2) on day 1 every 21 days.

We observed a higher incidence of grade 2-3 cumulative asthenia and worsening of performance status in the subgroup of patients who received cisplatin rather than carboplatin. Furthermore the postoperative mortality was 4% among patients treated with cisplatin compared to 0% among patients who received carboplatin in the induction chemotherapy regimen. We observed no difference in terms of disease control rate and progression free survival between the two treatment arms, while a longer overall survival (118 *versus* 66 weeks) was shown in patients treated with carboplatin rather than cisplatin. At the multivariate analysis, non-epithelial histology and cisplatin-based chemotherapy were associated to a worse prognosis. It is possible that a less aggressive chemotherapy regimen could improve the outcome of trimodality treatment, and allows second-line treatments to a higher proportion of patients. In our study, in fact, at the time of disease progression 37% of the patients previously treated with cisplatin received a second-line treatment, compared to 58% of the patients treated with carboplatin in the first-line.

Second line chemotherapy could have an impact on overall survival of mesothelioma patients, as already shown by Manegold and colleagues in the retrospective analysis of patients from the phase III study by Vogelzang in 2003 (Manegold et al., 2005). Another explanation for the longer survival in patients treated with carboplatin might be the higher number of sarcomatoid mesothelioma patients in the subgroup of patients treated with cisplatin.

As far as the doublet carboplatin and pemetrexed doublet concerns, another group recently compared that regimens to cisplatin plus pemetrexed in 54 malignant pleural mesothelioma patients (Emri et al., 2011).

Chemotherapy consisted of pemetrexed plus carboplatin in 34 patients and plus cisplatin in 20 patients; median number of cycles was 6. Surgery was performed in 41% of the study population, and radiotherapy in 29 (54%) patients.

Median overall survival in all the 54 patients was 16 months. When the authors compared overall survival in the two treatment subgroups, they observed a significantly longer survival in patients treated with carboplatin (20 months compared to 15 months in cisplatin-subgroup), while no difference in terms of time to relapse and response rate was observed between the two arms.

On the basis of those results, prospective randomized clinical trials should be designed to evaluate toxicity profile, response rate, survival data of different chemotherapy regimens in the neoadjuvant treatement of malignant mesothelioma patients.

6. Conclusion

Despite the improvement in diagnosis and treatment, malignant pleural mesothelioma patients still have a dismal prognosis, because of the low response rate to chemotherapy and the early relapses.

The integration of systemic and local treatments in the multimodality approach seemed to reduce local and distant recurrences, and subsequently to improve the overall survival of affected patients.

The optimal sequence of chemotherapy, radiotherapy and surgery has not been defined yet, even though trimodality protocols of neoadjuvant chemotherapy followed by extrapleural pneumonectomy and adjuvant radiotherapy achieved the best results, with overall survival longer than 20 months in selected patients.

The lack of a randomized study in this setting and the variability among the available phase II studies does not allow to draw any conclusion about the best treatment for mesothelioma patients. Furthermore, those studies evaluated data from selected patients who were eligible for trimodality treatment, subsequently introducing a bias in the final data analysis.

The role of EPP is still a matter of debate, and the recent results of the MARS trial suggests a potential role of a less invasive surgery, such as pleurectomy/decortication.

The optimal chemotherapy regimen in the induction phase is not defined, and prospective randomized studies assessing toxicity and survival data of different protocols should be designed.

To improve the response rate to chemotherapy regimen, new biologic agents should be introduced in the clinical practice, so that the best results in terms of tumor shrinkage and low toxicity could be achieved.

The optimal relationship between toxicity profile and clinical benefit should be investigated especially in the context of a trimodality approach, which implies a long-term treatment in patients who are often elderly and with impaired performance status.

Author details

Giulia Pasello and Adolfo Favaretto
Second Medical Oncology Dept., Istituto Oncologico Veneto, Italy

7. References

Buduhan, G., Menon, S., Aye, R., Louie, B., Mehta, V., & Vallières, E. (2009). Trimodality Therapy for Malignant Pleural Mesothelioma. *The Annals of Thoracic Surgery*, Vol.8, No.3, (September 2009), pp.870-876

Burdett, S., Stewart, L.A., & Rydzewska, L. (2006). A Systematic Review and Meta-analysis of the Literature: Chemotherapy and Surgery versus Surgery Alone in Non-small Cell Lung Cancer. *Journal of Thoracic Oncology*, Vol.1, No. 7, (September 2006), pp. 611-621, ISSN 1556-0864/06/0107-0611

Burdett, S., Stewart, L.A., & Rydzewska, L. (2007). Chemotherapy and surgery versus surgery alone in non-small cell lung cancer. *Cochrane database of systematic reviews*, Vol.18, No.3, (July 2007), CD 006157

Byrne, M.J., Davidson, J.A., Musk, A.W., Dewar, J., van Hazel, G., Buck, M., de Klerk, N.H., & Robinson, B.W. (1999). Cisplatin and gemcitabine treatment for malignant mesothelioma: a phase II study. *Journal of Clinical Oncology*, Vol.17, No 1, (January 1999), pp. 25-30.

Cao, C.Q., Yan, T.D., Bannon, P.G., & McCaughan, B.C. (2010). A systematic review of extrapleural pneumonectomy for malignant pleural mesothelioma. *Journal of Thoracic Oncology*, Vol.5, No.10, (October 2010), pp.1692-1703, ISSN 1556-0864/10/0510-1692

Castagneto, B., Zai, S., Dongiovanni, D., Muzio, A., Bretti, S., Numico, G., Botta, M., & Sinaccio, G. (2005). Cisplatin and gemcitabine in malignant pleural mesothelioma: a phase II study. *American Journal of Clinical Oncology*, Vol. 28, No. 3, (June 2005), pp. 223-226

Castagneto, B., Botta, M., Aitini, E., Spigno, F., Degiovanni, D., Alabiso, O., Serra, M., Muzio, A., Carbone, R., Buosi, R., Galbusera, V., Piccolini, E., Giaretto, L., Rebella, L., & Mencoboni,M. (2008). Phase II study of pemetrexed in combination with carboplatin in patients with malignant pleural mesothelioma (MPM). *Annals of Oncology*, Vol.19, No. 2, (February 2008), pp. 370-373

Ceresoli, G.L., Zucali, P.A., Favaretto, A.G., Grossi, F., Bidoli, P., Del Conte, G., Ceribelli, A., Bearz, A., Morenghi, E., Cavina, R., Marangolo, M., Parra, H.J., & Santoro, A. (2006). Phase II study of pemetrexed plus carboplatin in malignant pleural mesothelioma. *Journal of Clinical Oncology*, Vol. 24, No. 9, (March 2006), pp. 1443-1448

de Perrot, M., Feld, R., Cho, B.C.J., Bezjak, A., Anraku, M., Burkes, R., Roberts, H., Tsao, M.S., Leighl, N., Keshavjee, S., & Johnston, M.R. (2009). Trimodality Therapy With Induction Chemotherapy Followed by Extrapleural Pneumonectomy and Adjuvant High-Dose Hemithoracic Radiation for Malignant Pleural Mesothelioma. *Journal of Clinical Oncology*, Vol. 27, No. 9, (March 2009), pp. 1413-1418

Emri, S., Hurmuz, P., Kadilar, C., Cangir, A.K., Zorlu, F., Dogan, R., & Akyol, F. (2011). Pemetrexed-carboplatin doublets showed better mediab survival than pemetrexed-cisplatin in the treatment of Turkish malignant pleural mesothelioma patients. *Journal of Thoracic Oncology*, Vol. 6, No.6 (S2), (June 2011), pp. S 1671, Abtract n° P3.302

Favaretto, A.G., Aversa, S.M.L, Paccagnella, A., De Pangher Manzini, V., Palmisano, V., Oniga, F., Stefani, M., Rea, F., Bortolotti, L., Loreggian, L., & Monfardini, S. (2003). Gemcitabine Combined with Carboplatin in Patients with Malignant Pleural Mesothelioma. A Multicentric Phase II Study. *Cancer*, Vol. 97, No. 11, (June 2003), pp. 2791-2797.

Flores, R.M., Krug, L.M., Rosenzweig, K.E., Venkatraman, E., Vincent, A., Heelan, R., Akhurst, T., & Rusch, V.W. (2006). Induction Chemotherapy, Extrapleural Pneumonectomy, and Postoperative High-Dose Radiotherapy for LocallyAdvanced

Malignant Pleural Mesothelioma: A Phase II Trial. *Journal of Thoracic Oncology*. Vol. 1, No. 4, (May 2006), pp. 289-295, ISSN 1556-0864/06/0104-0289

Flores, R.M., Pass, H.I., Seshan, V.E., Dycoco, J., Zakowski, M., Carbone, M., Bains, M.S., & Rusch, V.W. (2008). Extrapleural pneumonectomy versus pleurectomy/decortication in the surgical management of malignant pleural mesothelioma: results in 663 patients. *Journal of Thoracic and Cardiovascular Surgery*, Vol. 135, No. 3, (March 2008), pp. 620-626

Kalmadi, S.R., Rankin, C., Kraut, M.J., Jacobs, A.D., Petrylak, D.P., Adelstein, D.J., Keohan, M.L., Taub, R.N., & Borden, E.C. (2008). Gemcitabine and cisplatin in unresectable malignant mesothelioma of the pleura: a phase II study of the Southwest Oncology Group (SWOG 9810). *Lung Cancer*, Vol. 60, No. 2, (May 2008), pp. 259-263

Krug, L.M., Pass, H.I., Rusch, V.W., Kindler, H.L., Sugarbaker, D.J., Rosenzweig, K.E., Flores, R., Friedberg, J.S., Pisters, K., Monberg, M., Obasaju, C.K., & Vogelzang, N.J. (2009). Multicenter Phase II Trial of Neoadjuvant Pemetrexed Plus Cisplatin Followed by Extrapleural Pneumonectomy and Radiation for Malignant Pleural Mesothelioma. *Journal of Clinical Oncology*, Vol. 27, No. 18, (June 2009), pp. 3007-3013

Manegold, C., Symanowski, J., Gatzemeier, U., Reck, M., von Pawel, J., Kortsik, C., Nackaerts, K., Lianes, P., & Vogelzang, N.J. (2005). Second-line (post-study) chemotherapy received by patients treated in the phase III trial of pemetrexed plus cisplatin versus cisplatin alone in malignant pleural mesothelioma. *Annals of Oncology*, Vol. 16, No. 6, (June 2005), pp. 923-927

Marinaccio, A., Binazzi, A., Cauzillo, G., Cavone, D., Zotti, R.D., Ferrante, P., Gennaro, V., Gorini, G., Menegozzo, M., Mensi, C., Merler, E., Mirabelli, D., Montanaro, F., Musti, M., Pannelli, F., Romanelli, A., Scarselli, A., & Tumino, R. (2007). Analysis of latency time and its determinants in asbestos related malignant mesothelioma cases of the Italian register. *European Journal of Cancer*, Vol. 43, No. 18, (December 2007), pp.2722-8.

Marulli, G., Rea, F., Nicotra, S., Favaretto, A.G., Perissinotto, E., Chizzolini, M., Vianello, A., & Braccioni, F. (2010). Effect of induction chemotherapy on lung function and exercise capacity in patients affected by malignant pleural mesothelioma. *European Journal of Cardiothoracic Surgery*, Vol. 37, No. 6, (June 2010), pp. 1464-1469.

Nowak, A., Byrne, M.J., Williamson, R., Ryan, G., Segal, A., Fielding, D., Mitchell, P., Musk, A.W., & Robinson, B.W. (2002). A multicentre phase II study of cisplatin and gemcitabine for malignant mesothelioma. *British Journal of Cancer*, Vol. 87, No. 5, (August 2002), pp. 491-496

Opitz, I., Kestenholz, P., Lardinois, D., Muller, M., Rousson, V., Schneiter, D., Stahel, R., & Weder, W. (2006). Incidence and management of complications after neoadjuvant chemotherapy followed by extrapleural pneumonectomy for malignant pleural mesothelioma. *European Journal of Cardiothoracic Surgery*, Vol. 29, No. 4, (April 2006), pp. 579-584

Pasello, G., Marulli, G., Nicotra, S., Rea, F., Loreggian, L., Bonanno, L., & Favaretto, A.G. (2011). Pemetrexed/Carboplatin or Pemetrexed/Cisplatin as first line treatment of malignant pleural mesotelioma (MPM): tolerability and response rate in operable patients. *Journal of Thoracic Oncology,* Vol. 6, No.6 (S2), (June 2011), pp. S1367, Abtract n° P3.297

Rea, F., Marulli, G., Bortolotti, L., Breda, C., Favaretto, A.G., Loreggian, L., & Sartori, F. (2007). Induction chemotherapy, extrapleural pneumonectomy (EPP) and adjuvant hemi-thoracic radiation in malignant pleural mesothelioma (MPM): Feasibility and results. *Lung Cancer,* Vol. 57, No. 1, pp. 87-95

Rea, F., Favaretto, A.G., Marulli, G., Spaggiari, L., De Pas, T.M., Ceribelli, A., Paccagnella, A., Crivellari, G., Russo, F., Ceccarelli, M., & Facciolo, F. (2011). *Journal of Clinical Oncology,* Vol. 29, Abstract 7090

Rice, D.C., Stevens, C.W., Correa, A.M., Vaporciyan, A.A., Tsao, A., Forster, K.M., Walsh, G.L., Swisher, S.G., Hofstetter, W.L., Mehran, R.J., Roth, J.A., Liao, Z., & Smythe, W.R. Outcomes after extrapleural pneumonectomy and intensity-modulated radiation therapy for malignant pleural mesothelioma. (2007) *Annals of Thoracic Surgery,* Vol. 84, No. 5, (November 2007), pp. 1692-1693

Rosell, R., Gòmez-Codina, J., Camps, C., Maestre, J., Padille, J., Canto, A., Mate, J.L., Li, S., Roig, J., Olazabal, A., Canela, M., Ariza, A., Skacel, Z., Morera-Prat, J., & Abad, A. (1994). A randomized trial comparing preoperative chemotherapy plus surgery with surgery alone in patients with non-small-cell lung cancer. *New England Journal of Medicine,* Vol. 330, No. 3, (January 1994), pp. 153-158

Roth, J.A., Fossella, F., Komaki, R., Ryan, M.B., Putnam, J.B.J., Lee, J.S., Dhingra, H., De Caro, L., Chasen, M., Mc Gavran, M., Atkinson, E.N., & Hong, W.K. (1994). A Randomized Trial Comparing Perioperative Chemotherapy and Surgery With Surgery Alone in Resectable Stage IIIA Non-Small-Cell Lung Cancer. *Journal of National Cancer Institute,* Vol. 86, No. 9, (May 1994), pp.673-680

Rusch, V.W., Rosenzweig, K., Venkatraman, E., Leon, L., Raben, A., Harrison, L., Bains, M.S., Downey, R.J., & Ginsberg R.J. (2001). A phase II trial of surgical resection and adjuvant high-dose hemithoracic radiation for malignant pleural mesothelioma. *Journal of Thoracic and Cardiovascular Surgery,* Vol. 122, No. 4, (October 2011), pp. 788-795

Song W.A., Zhou N.K., Wang W., Chu X.Y., Liang C.Y., Tian X.D., Guo J.T., Liu X., Liu Y., Dai W.M. Survival benefit of neoadjuvant chemotherapy in non-small cell lung cancer: an updated meta-analysis of 13 randomized control trials. *J Thorac Oncol.* Vol..5, No 4: pp. 510-6.

Stewart, D.J., Martin-Ucar, A.E., Edwards, J.G., West, K., & Waller, D.A. (2005). Extra-pleural pneumonectomy for malignant pleural mesothelioma: the risks of induction chemotherapy, right-sided procedures and prolonged operations. *European Journal of Cardio-thoracic Surgery,* Vol. 27, No. 3, (March 2005), pp. 373-378

Sugarbaker, D.J., Flores, R.M., Jaklitsch, M.T., Richards, W.J., Strauss, G.M., Corson, J.M., DeCAmp, M.M., Swanson, S.J., Bueno, R., Lukanich, J.M., Baldini, E.H., Mentzer, S.J. Resection margins, extrapleural nodal status, and cell type determine postoperative long-term survival in trimodality therapy of malignant pleural mesothelioma: results in 183 patients. (1999). *Journal of Thoracic and Cardiovascular Surgery,* Vol. 117, N0. 1, (January 1999), pp. 54-63

Treasure, T., Tan, C., Lang-Lazdunski, L., & Waller, D. (2006). The MARS trial: mesothelioma and radical surgery. *Interactive Cardiovascular and Thoracic Surgery,* Vol. 5, No. 1, (January 2006), pp.58-59

Treasure, T., Waller, D., Tan, C., Entwisle, J., O'Brien, M., O'Byrne, K., Thomas, G., Snee, M., Spicer, J., Landau, D., Lang-Lazdunski, L., Bliss, J., Peckitt, C., Rogers, S., Marriage, E., Coombes, G., Webster-Smitt, M., & Peto, J. (2009). The Mesothelioma and Radical Surgery Randomized Controlled Trial. The MARS feasibility study. *Journal of Thoracic Oncology,* Vol. 4, No. 10, (October 2009), pp. 1254-1258

Treasure, T., Lang-Lazdunski, L., Waller, D., Bliss, J.M., Tan, C., Entwisle, J., Snee, M., O'Brien, M., Thomas, G., Senan, S., O'Byrne, K., Kilburn, L.S., Spicer, J., Landau, D., Edwards, J., Coombes, G., Darlison, L., & Peto, J. (2011). Extra-pleural pneumonectomy versus no extra-pleural pneumonectomy for patients with malignant pleural mesothelioma: clinical outcomes of the Mesothelioma and Radical Surgery (MARS) randomised feasibility study. *Lancet Oncology,* Vol. 12, No. 8, (August 2011), pp. 763-772

Van Meerbeeck, J.P., Gaafar, R., Manegold, C., Van Klaveren, R.J., Van Marck, E.A., Vincent, M., Legrand, C., Bottomley, A., Debruyne, C., & Giaccone, G. (2005). Randomized phase III study of cisplatin with or without raltitrexed in patients with malignant pleural mesothelioma: an intergroup study of the European Organisation for Research and Treatment of Cancer Lung Cancer Group and the National Cancer Institute of Canada. *Journal of Clinical Oncology,* Vol. 23, No. 28, (October 2005), pp. 6881-6888

Van Schil, P.E., Bass, P., Gaafar, R., Maat, A.P., Van de Pol, M., Hasan, B., Klomp, H.M., Abdelrahman, A.M., Welch, J., & van Meerbeeck, J.P. (2010). Trimodality therapy for malignant pleural mesothelioma: results from an EORTC phase II multicentre trial. *European Respiratory Journal,* Vol. 36, No. 6, (June 2010), pp. 1362- 1369

Vogelzang, N.J., Rusthoven, J.J., Symanoski, J., Denham, C., Kaukel, E., Ruffie, P., Gatzemeier, U., Boyer, M., Emri, S., Manegold, C., Niyikiza, C. & Paoletti, P. (2003). Phase II Study of pemetrexed in combination with cisplatin versus cisplatin alone in patients with malignant pleural mesothelioma. *Journal of Clinical Oncology,* Vol. 21, No. 14, (July 2003), pp. 2636-2644

Weder, W., Kestenholz, P., Taverna, C., Bodis, S., Lardinois, D., Jerman, M., & Stahel, R. (2004). Neoadjuvant chemotherapy followed by extrapleural pneumonectomy in malignant pleural mesothelioma. *Journal of Clinical Oncology,* Vol. 22, No. 17, (September 2004), pp. 3451-3457

Weder, W., Stahel, R.A., Bernahrd, J., Bodis, S., Vogt, P., Ballabeni, P., Lardinois, D., Betticher, D., Schmid, R., Stupp, R., Ris, H.B., Jermann, M., Mingrone, W., Roth, A.D., & Spiliopoulos, A. (2007). Multicenter trial of neo-adjuvant chemotherapy followed by extrapleural pneumonectomy in malignant pleural mesothelioma. *Annals of Oncology*, Vol. 18, No. 7, (July 2007), pp.1196-1202